Living in the Moment

LIVING
in the
MOMENT

A Prescription for the Soul

GARY NULL, PhD

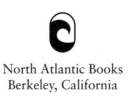

North Atlantic Books
Berkeley, California

Published by
North Atlantic Books
P.O. Box 12327
Berkeley, California 94712

Cover and book design © Ayelet Maida, A/M Studios
Printed in the United States of America

Living in the Moment: A Prescription for the Soul is sponsored by the Society for the Study of Native Arts and Sciences, a nonprofit educational corporation whose goals are to develop an educational and cross-cultural perspective linking various scientific, social, and artistic fields; to nurture a holistic view of arts, sciences, humanities, and healing; and to publish and distribute literature on the relationship of mind, body, and nature.

North Atlantic Books' publications are available through most bookstores. For further information, call 800-733-3000 or visit our website at www.north atlanticbooks.com.

Library of Congress Cataloging-in-Publication Data
Null, Gary.
  Living in the moment : a prescription for the soul / Gary Null.
    p. cm.
  ISBN 978-1-55643-763-2
  1. Self-help techniques. 2. Success. 3. Life. I. Title.
  BF632.N85 2008
  158—dc22

                                        2008013468

1 2 3 4 5 6 7 8 9 SHERIDAN 14 13 12 11 10 09 08

Acknowledgments

Over the years, I have had the privilege of engaging many of our world's most noteworthy thought leaders and visionaries in conversation. Some are the truly authentic voices addressing today's most pressing issues concerning our national and global crises and offering solutions to help us rise above the social apathy and spiritual malaise pervading our culture. There are too many people for me to name individually; however, during the preparation of *Living in the Moment*, several immediately stand out for their penetrating insight: Professor Emeritus Ralph Abraham at the University of California at Santa Cruz, Professor Morris Berman, Joan Borysenko, Dr. Lester Brown, Debbie Ford, Professor Ashok Gangadean at Haverford College, Dr. Jim Garrison at Wisdom University, Dr. Henry Grayson, Cheri Huber Roshi, Sandra Ingerman, Dr. Ervin Laszlo, Dr. Elizabet Sahtouris, Professor Tal Ben-Shahar at Harvard University, Dr. Alberto Villaldo, and Naomi Wolf.

I want to thank my radio show producer Richard Gale for engaging me in stimulating conversations about the boomer generation and its history, and about past and present spirituality. Our talks helped me to penetrate deeper levels of the topics addressed in this book. Also many thanks go to my staff and interns, in particular Betsy Ashley, Jay Gaynor, Doug Henderson, Damien Hickman, and Rachel Spratt.

Finally, a special appreciation goes to Anne Connolly for her excellent editorial work and to the folks at North Atlantic Books, in particular its founder, Richard Grossinger, and editor Emily Boyd for bringing *Living in the Moment* into print.

Contents

Introduction

While preparing for the final manuscript of the book you now hold in your hands, I attended the viewing of a wonderful documentary called *Young@Heart* by the British director Stephen Walker. The film follows a seven-week rehearsal schedule of a vocal chorus from a small Massachusetts community preparing for a new performance. The group of approximately two dozen singers travels around the country performing their own renditions of pop and rock songs from the 1960s, 1970s, and 1980s to packed halls.

What is significant about this particular chorus is that the singers' average age is eighty years old. The oldest is ninety-two. The film is often hilarious, yet at the same time it captures the pathos of our lives' fragility. Two of the chorus members pass away during the rehearsal period and the viewer is left feeling a deep sympathy for their loss. As a friend said about the film, it captures the contemporary impasse of a large portion of Americans who are simply waiting to die. Here is a group of seniors, their health ravaged by the adverse effects of the "standard American diet," who remain full of love, kindness, and a lust for life.

As a baby boomer sitting in the audience, I could not help but realize that in twenty years I could be in their situation. In fact, it conveys what my entire generation faces. Nevertheless, how often do we meet senior citizens doing something that is part of life's rejoicing and celebration, who fill their waiting days with such gusto and passion? Usually when we hear the word "seniors," we conjure images of old wrinkled people who are no longer productive members in our society. They live quiet, unobtrusive lives tucked away in gated communities somewhere in warmer climates. We are only reminded of their forgotten presence from television ads catering to the illnesses generally associated with our later years. Politically, we may hear their voices raised when Social Security or Medicare is threatened, or when their pensions lose money due to high-risk investment speculations. Otherwise, our seniors remain generally mute and abandoned in the shadows of irrelevancy.

Yet, as I watched *Young@Heart,* I realized seniors are still relevant. The enthusiastic applause from their audiences makes the singers feel they are individually greater than the composite of an age and illness. There are hidden qualities in each of us that solely want expression for their own sake and want to make the world a more pleasant place, and not in order to prove ourselves best or better than anyone else. These people are manifesting just that. Then I am reminded again of all the seniors who don't have a chorus to sing in or who don't have true friends who can share their company. And now we witness greater and greater numbers of seniors without sufficient money to sustain their bodies' proper nourishment, to pay for inflated drug costs, or to meet the rising fuel prices to keep their homes warm.

Parallel to the diminishing health and resources of our elders, I observe a growing segment of individuals among my generation—the children of our seniors' "Great Generation"—who have no sense of knowing when more is enough. Regardless of how far they have climbed on the social ladder or how above average their salaries are, they still take advantage of speculative gambling in hedge funds and quick revenue-generating investments in food commodities, fuel, and housing that have a direct impact on the lives of others. In fact, their exploitation of quick wealth opportunities hinders our seniors from the very things needed to raise them from an austere existence. In the first section of this book, "The Boomer Dilemma," I map out the historical terrain and the deep psychological underpinnings of the boomer generation that has brought America to the critical juncture we face today. Only by understanding the history of the boomers' development, their change in values, and what they have become in the twenty-first century, can we begin to shine a light on the actions necessary to bring about positive change.

Although I am embarrassed by some of the excuses of my generation, I am far more concerned about the future of our children and their children. It is for the benefit of future generations that I devote so much of my work in writing and directing controversial film documentaries about our social and institutional diseases and dis-ease. It is my opinion that we have yet to imagine the dire nightmare that looms ahead for the younger generation when it is their turn to receive the mantle of social and political governance left by the legacy of aging boomers.

Later that same evening, after watching *Young@Heart,* I returned to my office and watched the news. There were two horrid stories. One was about a group of twelve-year-old girls who filmed themselves beating up a classmate. The other story was about a student who attacked a teacher while the other classmates egged her on. Labeling these children as "monsters" completely misses the urgency of our social crises. It is far more important to realize that our children are the products of our generation's making. The real monsters are the institutions we have created, such as our failing political, educational, multimedia, medical, and religious systems, and the social values and motivations of the people who build and control them.

Several of our nation's courageous social critics, such as Morris Berman and Susan Jacoby, have—against much criticism—poignantly identified the growing anti-intellectualism and anti-rationalism ravaging all levels of American society. Our current president and his cabinet are exemplary cases and confirm Mark Twain's remark, "There are no common people except in the highest spheres of society." In 1965 approximately seventy-five percent of students entering college said they were pursuing higher education in order to discover something meaningful in life. In 2005 this same percentage of college students stated their goal was to become wealthy. In her book *The Age of American Unreason* Susan Jacoby notes that a recent National Science Foundation survey reported that one out of five Americans believe the sun revolves around the Earth. In addition, approximately half of young adults between the ages of eighteen and twenty-four are unable to locate Iraq on a map, and surprisingly, many are unable to find the United States.

There is something seriously wrong with this scenario and it forecasts a pending civic disaster on the future horizon. American culture is undergoing a collective, negative learning. The theory that each succeeding generation is actually regressing in its learning can be observed most clearly among today's college students. A recent study of 14,000 college students, across fifty American campuses, was published under the title "The Coming Crisis in Citizenship" by the Intercollegiate Studies Institute. The findings show that today's students are generally ignorant about American history and the institutions that govern our society. This finding didn't come as a great surprise to me; however, what I found alarming is that the students from the most elite universities—Yale, Johns Hopkins, Georgetown,

Brown, UC Berkeley, etc.—performed far below students at lesser-known colleges. In fact, the schools in the top ranking include some I have never heard of: Rhodes College, Grover City College, Calvin College, etc. This study suggests that the principles for rational and spiritual character development, which contribute greatly to the healthy moral development of a society, are less among students raised in privileged families. I believe one of the reasons is that many of our so-called brightest students today believe they are entitled to a prestigious education without having to achieve personal merit through hard work and effort. Yet this goes back to our present "culture of entitlement" that has raised them. Unfortunately, because our elite universities are held in such high esteem, we perpetuate a myth that these are the individuals best suited to run our institutions in the future.

On the flip side, faith in doctrinal laws dominates reason, and this is most evident in the continual growth of religious fundamentalist thinking. Our political arena is now one of the most fertile fields for faith-based missionary activity; politically motivated religion's underlying intention is to impose irrational laws upon human nature, with the ultimate goal to subvert American society at large. We are dressing ourselves in seventeenth-century garb—either as Puritans or Pirates—and charging blindly back to the past under a banner blazoned with "Forward." When we cease to find pleasure in entertaining our curiosities to learn about ourselves and the planet, the world again becomes flat. "No people," said Thomas Jefferson, "can be both ignorant and free."

The pursuit in frivolous, virtual entertainment devoid of any higher purpose offers nothing for authentic character development. Instead, it has increasingly numbed our senses and buried the innate gifts each of us is born with. When the mind and senses are no longer active and vital throughout the majority of a population, life in society is no longer worth living. It becomes *abyssus abyssum invocat,* "hell calling hell," which invokes the Dutch painter Bosch's residents in Dis wallowing gleefully in the chaos and confusion of distorted earthly delights. Until such a time arrives when we can be completely honest about how dysfunctional we have become, how empty of basic wisdom, we will continue our downward spiral.

Dr. Alberto Villaldo, a medical anthropologist and shaman, describes two co-existing universes: the universe of predators and the universe of creators. The world of corporate and political greed that we are witnessing today, the lack of ethics among investors and journalists, and the "me first" wealth-hungry values of our youth embody this predatory world. Alternatively, there is the world of creators, individuals who are gradually becoming the harbingers of a new culture based on enlightened reason, spiritual principles, and the restoration of social ethics based upon compassion, community, and personal responsibility for one's actions. One of the salient reasons for composing this book is to provide readers with some hard-learned inspiration to become a creator of harmony while living in our predatory culture. When we are able to become creators in a predatory society, and can remain in balance while doing so, we then have the capability for implementing genuine change.

The people who have the wisdom and courage to make the difficult decisions to implement real change, such as Ralph Nader, Ron Paul, and Dennis Kucinich, only received a small fraction of support from American voters. Instead, Democrats and Republicans equally display their support for the leaders most invested in corporate interests with an illusion that these individuals will bring about the real changes our times demand. The public neither has the patience nor vital curiosity to hear truth. Truth today is a sword of Damocles waved above their heads, and it is far easier to satisfy ourselves with blind faith in sound bites, catchy slogans, and the media's unlearned commentaries than to hear truths that compel us to make dramatic changes in our lives. And there can be no essential change from the current, popular political promises resounding through the air waves, such as additional government subsidies that court the public's demands for entitlement. While these perks may soothe some of our fears for a little while, they fail to address the fundamental infrastructure that is in dire need of repair. Today, the infrastructure that most requires mending is the infrastructure of consciousness, an infrastructure that needs to be cleansed of discredited and aging mythologies that continue to be enthroned as ontological and cosmological truths.

How did we reach this point in history when we can no longer discern authentic truth, when reason has been subverted by ignorance, where insecurity, instantaneous pleasures, and the rejection of personal responsibility for uplifting others have become the norm? This book is intended to be a mirror to help answer these questions. I hope we will perceive accurate reflections of what we have become. I hope we can equally observe the signs pointing to our authentic, true nature. This book is not meant to make us feel bad or angry about ourselves; rather its purpose is to bring a spiritual shock and awe that is so desperately needed today. The contemporary theologian Matthew Fox outlined succinctly the predicament of our personal responsibility toward ourselves and others. It is no longer sufficient for us to simply say, "Forgive us for we know not what we do." Rather, the mantra today should be, "Forgive us for we do not do what we know we should do." It is our apathy, complacency, and deep-seated fear of change that prevents us from taking that initial step forward to act as we ought to act.

No major social issue, such as poverty, the drugging of our nation and children, the war in Iraq and other global conflicts, and all the political, health, and educational crises, can change for the better until we as individuals change. Our systems for social and environmental sustainability are collapsing. We are utterly bankrupt, borrowing more than we actually have. Brutal reality television programs have become postmodern gladiatorial sports, sanctioned by our culture because they provide us with a means to escape our hectic, busy lives and to give us an excuse for not awakening from our cultural dream. The addict with collapsed veins who has no money to get his next fix is at a moment of great opportunity to allow healing to begin. But the needle and drug must go. And just like the addict, we must free ourselves from our addictions and face this road to recovery. It will not be pleasant. Contrary to the dictates of many popular pundits of supercilious, materialist spirituality—packaged as if lost secrets—it will not be an easy journey. Indeed, it will test us to the very core of our being.

I have attempted to outline clearly to everyone, regardless of the generation a person finds him or herself born into, all of the tools that are needed to reclaim our dignity and return as spiritually realized members of the human race. Each of us possesses qualities that are universal—love and compassion, kindness and nurturance—and these can generate harmony throughout the human community when they are brought to consciousness and acted upon. This book, therefore, is intended to provide and strengthen us with essential insights that will enable us to personally transform ourselves and thereby allow us to experience remarkable realizations of how extraordinary we really are.

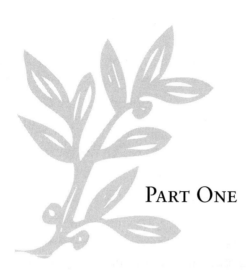

PART ONE

CHAPTER ONE

The Boomer Dilemma

Right now, millions of baby boomers are realizing they are no longer teenagers. For the next eighteen years, a line of approximately 78.2 million boomers will begin their exodus from middle age into senior citizen territory. Starting in 2010, almost eight thousand boomers will be turning sixty-five years old every day, or three hundred and thirty boomers every hour, according to the U.S. Census Bureau.

People in their forties and fifties are seeing wrinkles, gray hair, and bodies that are not what they used to be, and it is scaring them. They think of where their parents and elderly relatives were at the same age and remember them being old. Boomers don't feel prepared for that. Having devoted their middle-aged years to the frantic pursuit of securing a future for themselves, boomers are now waking up to the realization that the joys and vitality of life are passing them by.

From the 1960s, when boomers came of age and started entering the work force and finding their individual identity in society, to the present, boomers have fundamentally shaped American culture as we know it today. Every artist knows that there is a direct correlation between the mind and imagination of the artist and what he or she paints on canvas or sculpts in clay. An angry or depressed artist will produce works that emit those emotions to a viewer, and an artist full of joy and inner contentment will transmit a feeling of vibrancy and wholesome expansion. A similar parallel can be made to the values, lifestyles, pursuits, and attitudes of boomers and the world we now experience in the twenty-first century. It is important to understand this relationship to better appreciate and comprehend the boomer legacy—a trail that I now define an increasing alienation from and confusion about one's authentic self. Although their legacy includes important innovations in science, psychology, social reform, gender equality, and spirituality, it has likewise contributed to America's current cultural crisis and has shaped the nation into a populace that has lost its sense of civic virtue. By turning its back on the community- and family-based values that were the hallmark of boomer parents, the boomer generation is primarily responsible for our society's descent into social apathy, trivial pursuits, and unhealthy lifestyles.

I should make it clear that I am not suggesting that members of the "Greatest Generation," those born between 1911 and 1924 and who served in World War II, did not play a significant role in today's age of globalization, consumerism, and multinational corporate domination. Economists such as Milton Friedman, whose theories of free-market economics have essentially shaped the American economy since the Reagan presidency, when Alan Greenspan was first appointed as head of the Federal Reserve, belong to the Greatest Generation. However, the subsequent boomer presidents, Bill Clinton and George Bush, further strengthened the free-market economic system. Since the collapse of the Soviet Union, we have been experiencing the rapid proselytizing of a religion of consumerism—which underlies both the spiritual materialism of New Age thinking and the moralistic colonialism of right-wing fundamentalism in American religiosity—at the expense of once-vital industries and authentic spiritual altruism that made America the exemplar of the world during the aftermath of the Second World War.

The boomers are a generation that entered adulthood between the 1960s and the 1980s. They are a generation that wanted to have it all. Indeed, the baby boomers were the first generation that had been led to expect that they could have a superb education, a fulfilling career, a home with all the most recent appliances and gadgets, enjoyable relationships, and a family. While theoretically the boomers could have everything, practically, many could not. And many, although they attained all the prizes in the game plan, found that they could not achieve the happiness they had assumed would go with these prizes. They had worked too intensely, made (and in some cases also lost) a lot of money, and in the process burnt themselves out. Now, in the twenty-first century, we have millions of people who, if not completely demoralized, are walking around with a pervasive sense of unease and uncertainty. They have no energy. Their youthful idealism and rebellious expression, once this generation's historical signature, has nearly vanished. Now many boomers wish they could start all over.

The good news is that they can begin, if they're willing, a process of change and real transformation to renew the more positive ideals that once inspired their determination to address the wrongs, prejudices, and erroneous judgments in American society. Doing so requires actualizing one's self-awareness and synergizing this awareness with positive intentions and actions to improve the lives of others and their communities. One of the things I enjoy most is helping people reach a point in their lives where they're willing to make necessary changes, which is why I've written this book about the baby boomers' dilemma and our innate ability to live in the moment and recover what boomers have lost.

It has been wonderful to hear from people of all ages—from

teenagers to octogenarians and beyond—that my writing has made a difference in their lives. But in talking to members of the boomer generation I've been struck by the fact that so many are dissatisfied or have lost a sense of authentic purpose in their lives. These are some of the most well-educated, privileged, and savvy people in the nation. Why, in many cases, haven't they been able to use these assets to make necessary changes and find a measure of contentment? Some have understood intellectually the need to look within and repriorize their lives, but they've been unable to translate that understanding into meaningful change. They've conscientiously tried exercises such as meditating or going on spiritual or health retreats, but their outlooks have changed little. As members of this generation have left youth and advanced into middle age and beyond, many have a feeling of emptiness and continue to search for something they haven't found. The spiritual experiment for seeking self-discovery has been one of the characteristics of the boomer generation. One early statistic estimated that 42 percent of boomers left their families' religion or faith group; this is a significant figure and indicates how important the pursuit of self-expression has been among boomers. Their adventurous spirit in exploring alternative lifestyles, new models of health, different foreign philosophies and religions and art, is still influential today.

You might think it has been this way for every generation, that every generation undergoes difficulty in finding contentment and everyone has midlife crises. I don't think this is completely true. Boomers sacrificed the values and qualities that built America in exchange for lives of superficiality and a vision that focused attention on things that lack any essential meaning. For this reason, I find that this generation is having a particularly rough time recovering what it has lost.

The question is "why?" The baby boomers grew up during a

unique time in American history. They may have reached adulthood in the socially tumultuous late 1960s and 1970s, but people actually absorb their values in childhood, and for boomers that was the 1950s and early 1960s, a time when conventional values, seemingly reinforced by America's recent victory in World War II and by a growing industrial economy, were stronger than ever. Some conventional values were, and remain, good, but some assumptions and attitudes prevalent in those days were counterproductive to human fulfillment. My observation is that many boomers still carry around, unquestioningly and even unknowingly, attitudes and assumptions picked up during those years that are now causing them to make repeated mistakes in their personal choices.

Later I will outline some of the more critical mistakes that I see baby boomers commonly make. Although these are my observations, the important thing is the investigatory process and coming up with answers that are right for you.

At times I will address the boomer generation as a collective group; on other occasions I will address boomers as individuals, looking at the conditions of their inner lives. Each, however, mirrors the other. Our inner world shapes the conditions of our outer world. If we are angry at ourselves, we will project that anger onto others. The collective of all individual inner worlds—especially when they share the same values and follow the same regimens during their lives—shapes society as a whole. Although we frequently twist ourselves into thinking that our suffering, alienation, stress, and depression are solely our own, we also share these problems with everyone we meet, especially our children.

When we have the better part of our nation engulfed in a labyrinth of consumerism and ceaseless selfish pursuits for self-gratification, we ultimately end up with a society of citizens alienated from their authentic selves and from each other. It is my conviction that it is a moral imperative for boomers today to rekindle the spark that ignited their earlier civic and spiritual ideals and creative activism to reinstate a sense of sanity and balance in American culture. This was the underlying impetus for me to write this book. It is not important that you and I as boomers reap the rewards from our actions during our remaining days. Rather our motivation should be for the benefit of our children and their succeeding generations who will ultimately inherit the reins from us to govern and preserve American society in the not-so-distant future.

The Greatest Generation and Their Boomer Children

It is my belief that today's senior citizens—the members of the Greatest Generation—are the new "lost generation." They are the last of the American vanguard to have found meaning and purpose in the preservation and sustenance of the nuclear family, their communities, and nation. Before the arrival of boomer culture, preserving the health of these social units had always been a hallmark of American society. For the boomers' parent's generation, community defined a person's character. The Greatest Generation prided itself in what it had gained and what could be shared with others. Theirs was a culture of authentic altruism. It was all about interconnectedness and relishing the time spent with children, grandparents, and neighbors. Having food on the table surrounded by family, a steady job, a public education system for the children, clothing, and a house were all that was essential.

Stability is one of the keywords that best defines boomers' parents. One important area where they observed a pragmatic sense of stability was in the way they understood money and handled their finances. For them, a person's monetary power was determined by the amount of money saved rather than speculative assets. In other words, they perceived their financial worth in very concrete rather than illusory figures. Of course, credit cards did not exist then and any kind borrowing was generally the exception rather than the rule. This was a generation forced to live within its means, ensuring stability and continuity in their lives.

Not long ago, I had a chance to visit my old neighborhood in Parkersburg, West Virginia, a small city on the Ohio River. By today's standards of suburban sprawl, everything looked small and worn. While strolling along the familiar streets, once the play area for me and my friends, I heard two elderly voices call my name. It was Ms. Zoller and Ms. Croft, now in their eighties. They recognized me as if it were fifty years ago when they were young parents. I stopped to have a conversation and was amazed how they could recall minute details about my life growing up in Parkersburg. I asked them why they continued to live here and one of them replied, "Where are we supposed to live? This is all we know. Everyone else is gone but at least we know each other." I could not help realizing that both of these kind women lived so much in the past. Whenever they had an opportunity to speak about how things used to be, their faces would light up. At the same time, I could not help but feel these two ladies, like most senior citizens, feel their children have pushed American society far beyond their reach.

The work ethic has always been a part of American culture, and the Greatest Generation raised it to the highest standards. They believed that everything we wanted had to be earned through effort. Therefore, parents of boomers rarely gave free handouts to their teenage children, unless they were among the very wealthy. For example, if a boy wanted a new bicycle, his dad might say, "Okay, but I will only meet you half way. You have to perform chores around the house, or earn money cutting neighbors' lawns, and then you can have one." This was the kind of child-raising environment that transmitted a healthy merit-based work ethic to boomer children.

Then there came a brief time during the 1960s when the baby boom generation started to question their parents' work ethic altogether. Remember the "be-ins"? People were asking, in effect, "Why can't we sit around with flowers in our hair, and just be?" It may sound totally corny today, but I still think it was a darn good question. Unfortunately, it looks like most people have answered it, "Nope, it was a good idea at the time, but we can't just sit. Life's too complicated and demanding, so we've got to rush around like maniacs in our sport utility vehicles with our cell phones crammed to our ears. We've got to prepare for the next meeting, the next deal, the next activity, our children's future, our retirement. There's no time to just be."

Why is the boomer generation like that? Part of the reason is insecurity. The boomers were promised a golden future in the 1950s. At that time, everyone knew that with some study and hard work you could have all the basic essentials of the good life—the home, the car, and the family—most likely all would be financed by one salary from a company you could count on staying with for years. Two general assumptions were that most people would do better materially than their parents, and that society and the American Dream were by and large based on a meritocracy, so that the smarter you were and the harder you worked, the better you would succeed.

The change started in 1973 with the oil embargo. Suddenly there was a gasoline shortage, and talk about future severe energy shortages that would compromise our American way of life. As energy prices went up, so did inflation. And as the economic situation worsened, there no longer seemed to be a guarantee of the good life for everyone who worked hard. Women gained more access to the working world in the 1970s, which constituted progress in a real sense; the downside was that increasingly both members of a married couple had to work full-time just to keep the children fed.

In the 1980s, Reaganomics further eroded people's sense of security because the idea of a social safety net was questioned, and government programs were being weakened or dismantled. The prevailing ethos was that of "everyone for himself," so that even if you were doing well during that time you knew deep down that should things fall apart, you'd be on your own. It was no longer government's place to step in and help.

It was also during the 1980s that our tax system was changed in a way that furthered the stratification of economic classes, so that the "haves" wound up having more than the "have nots." While there might have been enough of the pie to go around if it was evenly divided, that was not going to happen, so the idea was to become one of the "have" group, whatever it took. The boomers had been made an implicit promise by the Greatest Generation—that with a little effort one could have a golden future—and if later years seemed to rescind this promise, they'd just have to work harder to keep the promise alive.

That's why becoming a workaholic seemed a sensible option to many. An extension of this thinking was that one's children should become workaholics too, to ensure their futures. The idea of competition infiltrated most areas of life, growing into the defining characteristic of our nation and society that it is today.

I do think that competition is a wonderful thing when you're competing against yourself. For instance, while most people who run the New York City marathon have no hope of beating the front-runners, anyone can compete with his or her own performance of the previous year and try for a personal best. That's a healthy kind of competition that helps people grow. But the kind of competition where you feel that you and your family have to grab yours before somebody else does is an unhealthy, mentally corrosive kind of competition. Many members of Generation X and the so-called Millennials—those in their twenties—define their lives around aggressive competition without regard for higher spiritual values in their present work or in the long-term results of their accomplishments. With the start of the downturn of the economy in 2007, more and more people are living pressurized, future-oriented lives that are based on the assumption that they're competing with the world.

The psychological consequence of always being possessed by the need to get ahead is that the mind becomes completely focused on satisfying its material desires and what the next move is to take the lead in the competitive game. The broader vision that enables us to perceive social and spiritual crises in our midst goes unnoticed. The problems around us are simply irrelevant because our self-gratification and need to get ahead in our consumer world takes precedence. Eventually, social and spiritual apathy set in.

During one of my radio programs in 2007, Dr. Jim Garrison, cofounder of the Gorbachev Foundation and president of Wisdom University, was a guest and we had very engaging dialogue about the aura of apathy that pervades America. According to Garrison and other historical scholars, the U.S. has been on a trajectory of growth and dominance on the world stage similar to that of other imperial powers throughout history. Today America stands at the apogee of what is known as the "imperial arc"—when wealth and power have been consolidated within a minority of elites (in our case, Washington and Wall Street)—the stage before imperial powers begin their gradual descent in status to becoming just another nation struggling among other nations. Or, in the worst case, the imperium decays into the dustbin of history. One requirement for building a vital civilization is a population's sense of civic virtue and willingness for self-sacrifice, generally known in American history as the Puritan ethic. If there were evident wrongs committed by the governing powers of the nation, citizens felt an obligation to speak, and regarded their effort to correct those wrongs worthwhile. The values of civic virtue and self-sacrifice were certainly an admirable trait of American society during World War II when the Greatest Generation transformed industry with innovative technology and science to come to the aid of its Allies in Europe and defend against the Japanese. Likewise, the boomers during the 1960s and early 1970s believed exerting their sense of civic virtue was worth the effort to bring an end to the Vietnam War.

But what happens when the consolidation of powers becomes so domineering—such as dictating what citizens should eat and purchase, what drugs will cure their illnesses, and how they should entertain themselves—is that people no longer feel they can effect any positive change in their community and nation, and question whether making an effort is even worth it. Instead they begin to exchange their sense of civic virtue for self-entitlement. I believe this accurately explains the overwhelming apathy throughout most of American society today. But even more interesting, especially when we acknowledge that this consolidation of wealth and power in Washington, Wall Street, and the corporatocracy is a product of baby boomers' addiction to competition, consumerism, and the pursuit of wealth, it also explains why such a large number of today's younger generation hold no higher ideals.

I don't think we have to strategize, scheme, and sacrifice for the future in ways that cut down on our enjoyment of the present. The flip side of excessive future-orientation is to discover happiness and joy in the present. Once we realize the moment as an endless fountain of happiness, contentment, and inspiration, we can regenerate our earlier ideals and imagination to find new solutions to the problems of our day.

Ideals and Imagination

In the early half of the twentieth century, the Swiss psychologist Carl Jung parted company from his mentor Sigmund Freud over their diverging theories of the definitions and roles of the imagination and the unconscious. For Freud, the unconscious was simply a waste basket of repressed emotions, which manifested as dreams and were signs, as it were, for earmarking conditioned learning and behavior. Jung, on the other hand, understood that the unconscious and the human gift of imagination possessed the keys to our creativity and our ability to see beyond the appearance of what reality presents to our senses. In his view, dreaming was a natural process inherent in the human being to heal the psyche. Our modern-day successors to Jung among boomers in humanistic and transpersonal psychologies have ushered in important transformations in the areas of alternative medicine and health. For example, the benefits of creative visualization for aiding immune responses to fight cancer and other debilitating diseases have now been researched in university and institutional laboratories and found effective. In addition, what is now called mind-body medicine has attributed many of its insights to Jung and other pioneers who explored the powers of the mind and imagination.

Imagination has been essential for many of the constructive cultural revolutions initiated by great humanitarians and visionaries. Countercultural movements, for better or worse, have always relied upon the powers of imagination to envision a lifestyle or society different than the status quo. Yet imagination needs to be tempered with reason to allow us to witness the healthy possibilities of our potential, to generate higher ideals to strive toward, and to inspire us with the motivations to improve ourselves and our communities. Imagination without reason and pragmatism easily goes awry because it lacks a grounded ideal for properly measuring the value of the images arising from the subconscious. Famous philosophers and psychologists have frequently warned of imagination's ability to slide into delusional perceptions about oneself and one's capabilities if not tempered by reason. The 1960s counterculture displayed both the best and worst of imagination's power. On the positive side, it contributed to youthful boomers speaking out against their parents' support or complacency toward the unjust war in Vietnam. It fueled the civil rights and feminist movements. During this time young adults also expressed their individual freedoms, freeing sexuality from their parents' puritan values and directing the eyes of the nation to the values of living a more simple lifestyle closer to nature. On the downside, the hippies' free reign of imagination, especially when stimulated by drugs, resulted in many bright, idealist boomers ruining their lives and facing tragic endings. Many more simply ceased to develop and mature, remaining as adolescents in aging bodies, and either succumbed to a variety of dysfunctions or abandoned their ideals to follow the siren's call for embracing a pseudo-American Dream in pursuit of wealth, power, and possessions.

One could argue that there were a lot of boomers who, while they didn't fully embrace the counterculture, identified with it somewhat. There were people like this on college campuses all over the country. But it's my feeling that these people had been so primed in the 1950s to respect the powers that be, that while they may have undertaken some token rebellion when it was the thing to do, later in life they fell back into the earlier mindset of letting others call the shots. On many campuses striking a hippie pose was the "in" thing to do, so that for many people whose hearts weren't fully into it, looking like a hippie was no more than an extension of the conformity of the 1950s.

Have you ever seen how elephants are trained in Indonesia for logging? Early in life, they are cross-chained with large chains that make it impossible to move or break free. Later on the chains are replaced with a simple little reed tethering the elephant to a tree. The elephant could break the reed with one yank, but doesn't. Early conditioning has created what seems like a real constraint, but isn't. Similarly, many people go through life limited not by real constraints but by illusions based on early conditioning. Like the elephants of Indonesia, they're being controlled not by real chains, but by the ghosts of earlier chains.

When the boomers were children, life and parenting supported the freedom of a child's imagination. As children we were able to pile up chairs and folding tables, toss blankets over them, and amuse ourselves with a fort or hideaway for hours on end. A flashlight in a dark room could be as entertaining as today's latest alien attack computer game. The former activates a healthy, creative imagination far more than the packaged illusion of the latter. There was of course less parental control during playtime, allowing kids to roam and play in the neighborhoods with friends, climb trees, and get filthy during their imaginative sojourns in parks, woods, and fields. Unlike today, the industrial complex of toy manufacturers and producers of children's television did not spin out endless illusions to occupy a child's imagination. There was a quality of realism in the toys of yesterday, or else toys were modeled off of fairy tales and fictional characters that possessed charm, innocence, beauty, and goodness. I am certain that the executives of children's entertainment firms never gathered groups of kids in a boardroom and allowed their imaginations to manifest grotesque monstrosities or the horde of Barbie dolls imitating Britney Spears and anorexic fashion models. These are solely the products of the baby boomers' desire to increase corporate profits, enhancing their own livelihoods at the expense of children's imaginations. The corporate shapers of children's entertainment, moreover, have taken advantage of the boomer parents' needs to have their children entertained while they indulge themselves in their hectic lives.

Every generation can be defined by its particular highs and lows. The highs comprise the unique gifts and *sitz em leben*—one's place in the greater scheme of life—defining a generation's true potential. The lows encompass all the negative conditions inflicted upon a generation by its parents and social and political institutions. It is fascinating to witness the interplay between generations during the course of recent American history. The Biblical account of the exodus from Egypt and the quest for a promised land can be reinterpreted as a myth for every generation. Each generation embarks on an exodus from the captivity of the social paradigm and values controlled by its parent's generation in order to create its own promised land. However, every generation's promised land in turn becomes an Egypt, a land of exile and alienation, for the succeeding generation. This cycle of generational sojourns through the social paradigms and expectations of preceding generations has been reenacted over and over. In every case a generation's ability to imagine a higher ideal has shaped its destiny. Here we are going to look at how the baby boomers' promised land has become a land of exile and alienation, full of disappointments, frustration, and anger, for their children. The danger I see is that the majority of today's younger generation might be the first in American history whose capacity to envision higher ideals for themselves has been smothered by the boomer generation's neglect to nurture positive values in its homes and communities. By the boomers' replacement of a viable work ethic with a culture of tension between competition and entitlement, young adults are now struggling to find a meaningful identity.

When imagination is snuffed out of a society, stasis and depression ensue. Mao Tse-tung's Communist agrarian revolution, which ultimately led to the Cultural Revolution and the atrocities committed by the Red Guard, is an extreme example. Mao and his comrade elites discerned everything in Chinese society as either black or white, permissible or banned. Many forms of traditional Chinese culture, entertainment, music, literature, art—all those activities that we generally associate with the imagination—were outlawed and replaced with political displays that didn't deviate from the ideal of Mao's socialist vision. Any product of the Western imagination was immediately suspect and regarded as an enemy of the revolution. All personal pursuits, even hobbies, were either sanctioned because they benefited the government's social ideology or were branded heretical, punishable by long prison internment or even death. For several decades, apart from entertaining their imaginations privately or in dreams, the Chinese population lived in a world empty of imagination and hence any valid spirituality, unable to manifest free expression in their personal lives.

During the past decades of the boomers' reign over American society, a very subtle form of subversion of the imagination has occurred. I do not want to suggest that this control over our children's imagination is intentional or even particularly conscious. What is important for us to realize is that the child's world today, defined and orchestrated by the boomers' social and corporate institutions— Hollywood, toy manufacturers, the computer and television entertainment industries—has been primarily defined by grown-ups, and this continues at the expense of children's freedom, their inherent personal gifts, and the power of their imaginations. There is no high ethical standard by which these industries operate other than competing for the population's attention to consume and consume more in order to sustain the illusion of a healthy, growing economy. The result has been the shaping of children's vital imagination into a hallucination, not by the innocence and free expression of the child, but by a bombardment of seductive images to mold children into loyal consumers for the future. This is not an expression of a healthy and positive imagination that reinforces spiritual values and free-thinking during a person's formative years.

Following the stage of innocence and preschool exploration of the world, children enter a school system to learn how to become productive members of society. How did the education system fail boomers, and in what way is the education system today, controlled by this generation, failing its children?

A critical shortcoming of a large segment of boomers has been their buying into a consumer-based corporatocracy and hence ignoring their generation's higher ideals for social and spiritual transformation. The pursuit of possessions and material comforts to provide a false sense of security has a psychologically numbing effect upon us. Things possess their own kind of gravitational pull when the mind and emotions become identified with them, often stronger than the lofty airiness of spiritual values and altruistic social goals. A fearful life preoccupied with its welfare and security in the future is a life of constant struggle, competition and turmoil. The ancient Greek two-faced goddess Hecate, also known as Kore, portrays the dual sides of life experience. In the Greek Mysteries she was regarded as an image of the world soul, the energy behind all that lives and breathes. On the one hand, when our mind is immersed in the density of possessions and consumed with the pursuit of finding security in things and inane activities, Hecate's face appears wrathful. It indicates that when we turn our attention only toward how we can satisfy our gross physical senses, the world becomes a realm of constant struggle and unnecessary suffering. Alternatively, when we place our attention on higher values, on how we can improve ourselves, manifest our full potential, and benefit the lives of others, Hecate's other face appears caring and benefic. Life then flows effortlessly. For the Greeks, Hecate's face of joy embodies what sages have referred to as the contemplative life, a life with opened eyes; the life I refer to as living in the moment.

Another instructive image about possessions' psychological burden is found in the famous ancient poem, "The Hymn of the Pearl" in the early apocryphal text *The Acts of Thomas,* which influenced the wonderful German film *Wings of Desire* by Wim Wenders. The poem is an excellent analogy for how we lose our bearings in life when we become overly attached to the accumulation of possessions and forget our spiritual identity and higher values.

The hymn is about a king who sends his boy to recover a pearl guarded by a serpent in the sea. During his sojourn, the boy enters a country renowned for its obsessive pursuit of possessions and its self-indulgence and superficial pleasures, which he had earlier been warned about. The boy is quickly seduced by the citizens' lifestyle of mindless, selfish trivialities and is lulled into forgetfulness about his true origins as the son of a great king. He becomes simply another citizen, void of any unique identity, just another obedient servant of the country's ruler. Eventually a messenger delivers him a letter from his father. The letter awakens his memory to who he truly is, and he continues on his journey to recover the pearl.

The story is a compelling portrait of young adults' immersion in boomer culture. The question is: Where are the parents who will deliver the letter reminding their children of their authentic self and purpose on Earth?

Boredom prevents us from actualizing our true potential; in fact, it makes us forget we even have one. We might engage ourselves in endless activities and busyness, but this only gives us a superficial feeling that we are not bored. Just like the boy in the hymn who forgets his royal heritage, we inadvertently become servants to whatever the social system tells us. We lose sight of the precious pearl awaiting us, a symbol of our authentic self and true potential, which brings joy, peace, and happiness into our lives. Yet we have become conditioned from childhood to be experts in boredom, and our educational system has been the supreme guru in initiating us into a society of mediocrity, empty of spiritual value and fulfillment.

The serious failures of today's education system began before the baby boomers and the World War II generation. The origins of the system we have inherited today can be traced back to America's towering early twentieth-century industrialists: Andrew Carnegie, John D. Rockefeller, J. P. Morgan, and Henry Ford. In 1924, the ever-insightful social critic and satirist H. L. Mencken wrote that the purpose of public education during his time was not

> to fill the young of the species with knowledge and awaken their intelligence.... Nothing could be further from the truth. The aim ... is simply to reduce as many individuals as possible to the same safe level, to breed and train a standardized citizenry, to put down dissent and originality. That is the aim in the United States, and that is the aim everywhere else.

In his excellent expose on the origins of modern education, *The Underground History of American Education*, John Taylor Gatto identifies three fundamental principles that had defined the best of American education in the past: 1) to develop good, caring people,

2) to develop good citizens in the community, and 3) to make every student discover their higher, unique purpose and to guide them in developing it to its maximum. These principles, in fact, mirror the aspirations of the nation's founding fathers, such as Jefferson and Franklin, who envisioned a robust, discerning, and enlightened America.

However, with the advent of the industrialists mentioned above and others such as the founder of the Social Efficiency Movement, Frederick Winslow Taylor, in the 1910s these principles were replaced with a single goal: since children were seen as a "human resource," education's directive became to prepare students to find their place in the industrial world. This goal was not only the vision of the industrial leaders, but was also adopted into American politics in the White House. Gatto documents these words of Woodrow Wilson before he became president, "We want one class of persons to have a liberal education, and we want another class of persons, a very much larger class, of necessity, in every society, to forgo the privileges of a liberal education and fit themselves to perform specific difficult manual tasks." It is my belief that this perversion of public education's role into producing bored workers and consumers in the future continues today in a modified manner. The difference is that sitting at a machinist's bench has been replaced with sitting in a corporate cubicle with a computer.

We might remember that there was a single fear that utterly petrified industrial moguls like the Carnegies and Rockefellers; that is, the threat of a workers' revolt to topple their positions of power and control over vast wealth, power, and influence as they had witnessed with the Bolshevik Revolution in Czarist Russia and the rise of unions in industrial Europe. For this reason, the American power elite during the early twentieth century needed to reshape all American institutions—education, medicine, universities, management, et cetera—to assure that the population was isolated from independent, free-thinking influences in order to prevent their imaginations from entertaining higher ideals and visions that might threaten the dominant social paradigm. Few Americans know that the current mass public education system that we have today was originally adopted from a model developed in Prussia, which had been proven to produce bored, mediocre minds who would surrender themselves to their allotted place in society without challenging authority. The result has been that every generation has since removed another nutrient from public education until today we have Wonder Bread schooling—colorless, bland, tasteless, and void of any authentic nutritional value for human consumption whatsoever.

Baby boomers have succeeded in further dumbing down education by making standardized testing a reductionist science. Perhaps unbeknownst to them, it has been a superb tactic ensuring that the fire of passion and imagination is finally extinguished in their children. Replacing the earlier principle of identifying each student's unique talents and developing them to a higher and more inspired level, standardized testing is doing little more than providing students with the bare of essentials, equivalent to teaching every child how to go to the bathroom and to brush their teeth on their own. The result is a generation, now in their twenties and thirties, who are extremely intelligent, able to recognize the lies and hypocrisies of boomers' corporate, political America, and that of all its many institutions including the faith communities. However, instead of possessing ideals to carry society to a higher level of realization, most are spiritually adrift and extremely distrustful of everyone except a close circle of friends. Worse, because their imaginations have been severely repressed as children, both at home and in school, they are a generation wandering in a desert without any authentic vision for a life other than competing for money, dominance, and indulging in ceaseless entertainment. And what happens when maturing youth lack the imagination to create a noble ideal to strive for? They expect entitlements and rewards for simply inhabiting a body and being in a culture that has lost its ethical bearings and whose only purpose is endless consumption.

Baby boomers' commitment to corporate interests has also ensured that our children remain not only mentally handicapped but also physically unhealthy. Large revenue-generating food services in public schools provide children with the worst imaginable foods for human consumption. We have allowed companies to make soft drinks—heavily concentrated with sugar, caffeine, and phosphoric acid (equivalent to gargling with battery acid)—readily available throughout schools. It is well known that junk food disturbs our mental faculties and can lead to depression because it offers no essential nutrients for the brain. Consequently, children are bouncing off walls in classrooms and acting unruly and aggressive toward each other. Their mental capacity to concentrate on any given topic or task for an extended period of time is limited. Change the diet of children and we will witness a decrease in the seeming ADD and ADHD epidemic. The boomer parents who permitted businesses and vested interests in educational organizations to toxify their children will no doubt proclaim innocence. In response I am reminded of a modern Sufi saying, "Innocence without wisdom is ignorance; wisdom without innocence is arrogance."

Although this might appear a bleak scenario, we should remind ourselves that while imagination can be repressed, it does not disappear altogether. Every person possesses latent visionary qualities and ideals that can be actualized. Imagination is inherent in the human being and I have hope that the children and grandchildren of baby boomers will rekindle their imaginations and act upon their ideals in a positive manner. After the collapse of the Soviet Union and the

opening of China to Western ideas and values, there was a burgeoning of spiritual idealism that was never completely absent but had
remained dormant during the decades of Communist ideological
oppression. But I have little hope for anything truly constructive,
authentic, and transformative being actualized en masse by baby
boomers as they prepare for retirement in gated communities or struggle against the inevitability of age while they spend the rest of their
lives in boredom.

Boomers do have the opportunity, however, to reinvent themselves by reinvesting in the development of their inner lives in order
to improve the quality of their outer lives as well as the lives of their
children and friends. It is never too late. As children, boomers were
not consciously encouraged to develop their inner lives. Although
daydreaming and seeing little invisible people and playmates might
have been cute, we were told it was just fantasy and it would not
benefit us. It wouldn't put food on the table or get us a home or the
man or woman we would marry later. Many boomers take their criticism toward the inner life of their children even further—denying
its usefulness outright. Children and teenagers are told repeatedly—
not just by parents but also by the entire multimedia culture—that
they should focus only on the outer world because that is where success and happiness will be achieved. Consequently, our inner lives
are impoverished. With few exceptions, churches and faith groups
have completely failed to encourage the inner life although traditionally this was spirituality's ultimate task. It has always been the
premise of authentic spiritual paths that the toxicity we experience
in the outer social world is but a reflection and manifestation of the
toxicity within ourselves.

One of the greatest teachers for helping us redeem ourselves for
having ignored and even denigrated our inner life at times, is nature.
If we frequent settings outdoors—even if it is simply an urban park

with trees and the sounds of birds—we can reconnect with the deeper world inside us. The sun is always present wherever we are. We come in contact with water daily, and with the greenery of the plant kingdom. Green is also the color of internal healing in many traditional healing and spiritual paths. Once we can realize the preciousness of life and our planet, we will revitalize our appreciation for the preciousness of our own lives. Only then can boomers transform aging into saging and begin mentoring the generations drawing closer to replace them.

Neo-patriotism

Before September 11, 2001, globalization was already a key concept on the minds of many people around the world. There were best-selling books by authors taking sides in debating globalization's merits. For example, *New York Times* columnist Thomas Friedman has been a rabid supporter of American corporate interests enveloping the planet, while the Nobel Prize laureate in economics, Joseph Stiglitz, has been one of globalization's most outspoken critics. The news frequently reported on demonstrations all over the world against the captains steering globalization: institutions such as the World Bank and IMF, the World Trade Organization, and elite multinational corporation clubs like the World Economic Forum.

Globalization is a highly complex phenomenon and difficult to wrap our minds around but in its present state it is a baby boomer creation for finding ways for Americans and citizens of other countries to consume more and more. One thing we can probably agree upon is that almost everyone today feels like the planet is a much smaller place than it was fifteen or twenty years ago. Regardless of globalization's rights and wrongs—and there are many of each— the emergence of a planetary consciousness where every person is both a citizen of a nation and a resident of the planet has gradually taken root. Today, to be a strict isolationist is to be mentally alienated from the modern world. However, after the attack on the World Trade Center, this global awareness seemed to be placed on hold as Americans fell back into a patriotic, nationalist mindset. Even in our age of globalization, Americans generally still hold a distorted perception about the world, other nations and cultures. Among citizens in the developed world, Americans, in terms of percentage of the population, hold the fewest passports. As a nation, we have seen less of the world than other countries have. Even among those who have traveled outside America's boundaries, their international experience is usually limited to tourist watering holes like Cancun, Barcelona, or Miami, to resorts that can be found anywhere around the world. Of course, if you live in the Netherlands, for example, you would only have to drive a couple hours to be in a new country with a different language, a different cuisine and culture, and a different political climate and customs. Consequently, Europeans are far more sensitive to the diversity of the human community. For this reason we still find a remnant of statesmanship among some European leaders whereas in America statesmanship is all but extinct.

I find it quite fascinating to observe how the new fervent nationalism—a belief that "my country is best" against all others—reflects a fundamental belief held by the parents of boomers. However, the differences between the nationalism of the Greatest Generation and our current boomer nationalism are immense. The pride the Greatest Generation had for the nation was authentic and reflected a reality shared by other nations. America was loved around the world for its role in defeating the aggressions of Nazi Germany and Japan. The industriousness of the American worker and our innovations in almost all scientific disciplines were held as exemplars for other nations to emulate. The United States back then was often considered the best country in the world—this is certainly what boomer children were taught in school. Today, people may make fun of multiculturalism and the political correctness thereof, but it's still constructive to question the old belief in "my country, right or wrong." In fact, it is more important to hold this belief accountable today than ever before.

One of globalization's positive contributions has been providing us with greater exposure to other cultures and the possibilities to learn from them. The baby boomer generation helped begin this process with the counterculture and activism of the late 1960s. The boomers, as a group, began the burst in foreign travel, with their desire to experience all the world had to offer. Many immersed themselves in the lifestyles of the different cultures they visited, and in turn introduced foreign cuisines, child-rearing practices, alternative medical modalities, and techniques in self-development and spirituality that have become readily available throughout America.

To illustrate one simple example with child-rearing practices, anyone carrying a baby around strapped to their chest or back during the 1950s would have been considered out of their mind. But this is precisely what mothers throughout Africa and South America have done for thousands of years. These cultures knew that by keeping the infant close to your body, even while you work and go about your daily chores, the child remains content and happy. Americans, to their credit, caught on. Boomers also began exploring prolonged breastfeeding and natural childbirth, which in the 1950s were the kinds of things that only so-called primitive people did. Or look at the "family bed" concept, where everyone—parents, babies, and young children sleep together, as they do in many Native American and other indigenous cultures. This is not what we've traditionally been told is right in this country, but there are increasing numbers of psychologists today propounding the family bed concept, and more American families are practicing it.

Although there was a time when Americans opened themselves to learning about the cultural richness and wisdom of foreign societies, I believe we have witnessed the diminishing of this ethic since 9/11. There has been a return to the belief that "America is best" and a renewed support in Wilsonian U.S. intervention in other parts of the world, with a goal of protecting our nation's interests and well-being under the guise of spreading democracy. At home, particularly amongst the boomers on the Christian far-right, this is being interpreted as a blessing of providence under the banner of a new Manifest Destiny, which is completely alien to the teachings of America's founding fathers. However, other economies have already rapidly overtaken us; European nations have far better foreign policy relations with developing countries, and the EU and Japan are better protecting their citizens from pesticides, genetically modified foods, and harmful toxic chemicals in common household products. I heard from a friend among a group of American global activists who met with members of the Brazilian elite during the World Social Forum in Brazil—a movement to counter the huge multinational corporate interests held by the World Economic Forum—that these wealthy family heads said, "We no longer want our children to go to college in the U.S. It isn't that your education isn't excellent. It is. However, we don't want our children exposed to your current values and attitudes toward life. Instead, we plan to send our children to universities in Europe, Australia, or Japan." It used to be the case that privileged families all around the world wanted to enroll their children in American universities because our higher education was held in such high regard. But today, tell any American that European education might be better and might provide a healthier environment for learning than in the U.S. and you will receive a tongue thrashing. The belief in America's past laurels continues to determine the way we perceive ourselves, our nation, and the world.

It's important to understand that the issue of horizon-broadening goes beyond interest in other cultures. At a deeper level, if people aren't willing to look at their cultural assumptions, they aren't going to be willing to look at any of their assumptions about life. They're just going to plod through their days unquestioningly, following down the same narrow path that they've been following for years and that others have followed before them, stuck in the same old ruts that are getting deeper and deeper all the time. Were I to suggest getting off this path, and getting on a wider, fresher, more scenic one, these people are going to give me reasons why making a change is not practical. The problem is that there can be no essential learning when the mind is closed. There are people who refuse to make even small mental changes in order to expand their outlook on life. This is a shame because with the world as our classroom, there is so much we can learn.

You can go to Spain and see how they don't have to say "Let's do lunch" there, because they "do lunch" every day with their families, enjoying a relaxed main meal for at least an hour. It keeps family ties strong, and is better for the digestion than our custom of eating our largest meal in the evening.

You can go to Hungary or Turkey and observe how young people there are guided by their elders through the difficult passages from childhood to adolescence to adulthood. Guidance there is not just something you get from an office in school. In these other cultures, aging is understood as process of becoming wiser and elders continue to take on the role of guiding the youth in the ways of wise living.

You can talk to Native Americans about what the concept of nature means to them. It's a sacred part of everyday life, not merely some frill to be enjoyed on weekends, or a force to be controlled, owned, erased, or put on exhibit. Instead, nature is perceived as a

living entity and as the fundamental source of our sustenance. Therefore, they believe it is the duty of people to preserve the environment.

I could go on, touching upon dozens of cultures, but it all boils
down to this: If you're open to the world and avoid prejudging it,
the world will open up a wealth of useful knowledge and perspectives
for you. This is true on every level of experience.

A friend of mine has an interesting story about how prejudging
doesn't work:

> Up until my late thirties, I'd just sort of assumed that you
> were friends with people in your own age group who were
> going through roughly the same stage of life you were. There
> was a woman in my neighborhood whom I only began talk-
> ing to because we'd both gotten involved in a local political
> struggle to save trees in a park. It seems silly now, but I found
> her a little scary at first because she was in her seventies, her
> skin was all wrinkly, and her eyes were slightly crossed. When
> I saw her, my first reaction was "strange." She'd never had
> kids, and was not the type to pretend interest in other people.
>
> Here's what I discovered: I had more in common with this
> woman than with a lot of the moms my age. She truly cared
> about the local park and its trees because, like me, she liked
> to walk on a trail there. She had the kind of spirit, energy,
> and interest in the world that some people call youthful, but
> that is really ageless. When I talked with her it was like being
> back in the exciting world of a college campus, where exchang-
> ing real ideas was an important part of conversing. To tell the
> truth, getting together with her was a lot more stimulating
> than talking with other mothers about the cutoff date for
> kindergarten. But I never would've suspected this at first glance.

I would like to share another example of this principle. It might not always be a person's intellect or what they do that attracts us. Sometimes it can just be a person's being and presence. The producer of my radio program has traveled extensively around the world and has spent time with many notable people—the Dalai Lama, Mother Teresa, Mikhail Gorbachev, Jane Goodall, and others, but once when were talking, he said that when people ask him who the most inspiring person he ever met was, only one person immediately comes to mind. It happened to be a middle-aged woman with advanced leprosy living in an old graveyard in New Delhi. He said that he would visit her in her tiny hut, which had a tombstone for one wall, and sit there and watch her make tea for him. She owned almost nothing; she was a social outcast, considered utterly impure by Indian society. But as he watched her balance the kettle over the burning cow dung in a pit in the clay ground, pouring the tea into cups with her fingerless hands, he saw that she made every movement with perfect grace. She moved about on stubbed legs like a ballerina, her eyes were caring, and her presence full of peace. He said he learned more about the dignity and potential inherent in a human being from the silent presence of this woman than from any of the other better-known teachers he studied with.

So we need to venture outside of our judgments, constrained beliefs, and compartmentalized lives to open up to experience. What if you were to simply refrain from prejudging everything you think about? You wouldn't reject all the places you hear negative things about. You wouldn't dismiss people until you got the chance to know them. Think of how much more of the world you'd be open to experiencing.

You can never change anyone in life (not that you have the right to anyway); if you think you're smart enough to change someone, think again. We live in a world of multiple realities. There is a place for everyone. If you don't accept other people's realities, they may close off a side of themselves. All you are doing then is accepting someone who has changed superficially to be accepted. As a result, you never expand your outlook on life, and you pay a price for that. If you can accept a person who is completely different from you, and honor those differences, you will have the opportunity to build a rich relationship. The differences can enhance you as much as (or more than) what you have in common does.

We have come to accept knowledge as growth, that all we need is more new information to make wise decisions. If we have enough facts and equations, then somehow a solution to a problem will automatically become clearer to us. I would challenge this assumption. First, we can ask ourselves whether the world is really better due to all the information we have piled up. Why do so few people have healthy, functioning lives? It certainly has not been because we are deficient in information. Therefore, consuming facts and information has its limits.

There has been much written about living in the new Information Age. Boomers have been the masters of information gathering and hoarding. Our present age is really the boomer era that was ushered into the lives of Americans with the advent of the personal computer, when our ability to mine vast collections of data and facts for whatever exploitive purpose took off. The endless acquisition of information is in many respects just another expression of the boomers' consumer society. It makes us feel better if we think we know more. The consequence has been that we have many intelligent and knowledgeable boomers but the authentic wisdom necessary for applying this information is at poverty levels. Although we are not short on information, we have become seriously deficient in developing new perspectives and new ways of framing problems that leave old beliefs, prejudices, and bigotry behind.

Ultimately, the information we acquire must coincide with universal truths. For example, if we are conditioned not to trust someone because of prejudiced and erroneous information we read or hear about, perhaps regarding a person's nationality or religion, on the surface we may believe this to be true, but our inner consciousness knows it to be a lie. It is not a universal honesty. You have to match your individual beliefs to universal truths. To do this, you must frequently take a big step outside of your belief system. To understand what is universal, we have to look at the consequences of our beliefs. That which honors life is universally true. No one has the right to take another life, for instance. And no one has the right to dishonor anyone.

Some people see what's right for them personally, and then they stop their thinking right there. I interviewed some boomers who worked in a company that made pesticides that were banned in the United States but sold legally overseas. I found out that hundreds of thousands of pesticide poisonings, and thousands of deaths from those poisons, had occurred in China and other countries. I asked these people, "Is it right for you to be working in a company that makes a product that hurts people in another country?" Their answer, almost uniformly, was, "I'm not doing anything wrong. I'm just making a living." They were making a living by taking other lives, but that didn't seem to matter.

People do not feel connected to their extended reality. That's why a bomb maker doesn't think about where the bomb is going to be used. Imagine working in a factory that makes land mines. Every day, children throughout the world are getting their limbs blown off because someone planted a mine. There are millions of these mines, and even decades after so many wars have ended, responsibility and efforts at top levels to cease landmine production fall short. I could never work in a factory where I knew that something was being made that could destroy a human life. I could not work for mega-corporations like Bechtel and Halliburton that destroy the infra-structure and resources of other communities and nations in the name of Western development and globalization. When boomers were coming of age they held more value in living by universal truths, but some of them have forgotten this. So we should never forget that everything we do extends to others. This is why it is so necessary for us to see the larger reality that affects us all.

The people in control of the nation and economy want you to spend what you don't have on what you don't need. So they get you to believe you have to maintain an image, and this becomes part of the American Dream. But the part of the American Dream they don't tell you about is the nightmare of the payments that you can't meet, and the imbalance in your own life as you devote more time to work and less to family, friends, community, and outside interests. One morning you wake up thinking, "We have everything we're sup-posed to have. Why are we so dysfunctional?"

Imagine how devastating it would be for the people in power if you stopped buying. They wouldn't like it, but you would have the freedom to do more. If you wanted to go on a long trip with your family, or alone, you could. If you wanted to go to other countries and enjoy different cultures, you could. For some people interna-tional travel can initiate an expansion of their horizons, enabling them to identify as a citizen of the earth instead of just a patriot of a given country. If you wanted more quiet time for meditation, you could work that into your life. You'd be able to build your life around what is essential to you.

Letting go of the American Dream involves a new mindset. It means that we have to content ourselves without many of the toys we are addicted to. It also means learning to feel good about yourself in the face of judgments from others. If you are a fifty-year-old with a college degree who gives up a job and house and moves to a remote area to start a new life, you are going to be considered irresponsible by most people. You must realize that you are being responsive to your own needs, and that that is more important than living just for others. After all, you can't live this day over. Until you make your time valuable, it is used only for spending. You are merely a tool of the multinational corporations. Once you reorient yourself, you do not belong to anyone else's belief system and you are free to go wherever you want to go and do whatever you want to do. Honor your time by your own standards, not by someone else's.

Religious and Spiritual Materialism

With all of my discussion about the limits of our society's overindulgence in consumerism and competition, and the loss of deeper spiritual values associated with nurturing the wisdom found in our inner lives, someone might say, "Wait a minute, Gary! America is the most religious nation in the developed world. As of early 2002, surveys by respectable research groups, such as the Pew Charitable Trusts and the Barna Research Group, estimate that 86 percent of American citizens report their affiliation with a religious faith—whether orthodox, traditional, or unconventional. So how can you say there is a substantial loss of spiritual values in America today?"

My answer is quite simple. Adhering to a belief system is not the same as living with the deeper awareness about the essential meaning of that belief's values in one's life. A belief system is just that: a system. It is a system that stands alongside or in opposition to other systems. And history shows that all systems change. Since systems are edifices of human imagination, all systems are impermanent. If Christians in the twenty-first century could transport themselves to the origins of Christianity in Palestine two thousand years ago, they would likely not fully relate to the faith practiced at that time. Therefore, it is important to realize that belief systems, although powerful and capable of exerting great influence over a society, are still by definition subject to change. Nor does a religious system necessarily impart universal values upon its members. For example, there are many devout Christians, Jews, and Muslims—in America and abroad—thoroughly devoted to their respective belief systems, who are eager to bomb each other off the face of the earth.

Some of today's faith communities have become places of refuge for many boomers, as well as for members of other generations, who have arrived at the realization that the domineering edifices of American society—in politics, finance, business, healthcare, education, et cetera—are impersonal and unsupportive of community building today. The surge into more orthodox religions, particularly evangelical Christianity, is not necessarily about a person's personal desire to embark upon a path of self-discovery as much as it is about finding human acceptance and a sense of community in a culture that has turned cold and has left its citizens to fend for ourselves. Many boomers with hectic lives and insufficient time to spend with their children and families have recognized this need. But instead of taking it upon themselves to make the necessary lifestyle changes to accommodate other family members, they have found faith communities to be the answer to their needs and prayers.

Conventional religion is not the only major expression of faith in American culture that boomers have participated in. There is also an alternative belief system that has burgeoned into citizens' lives via mass media and popular self-empowerment gurus, which falls under the umbrella term of the New Age.

The recent success of *The Secret,* both the book and its subsequent film, is indicative of a pervasive outlook that is particularly strong among baby boomers. The essential premise of *The Secret* is that if we put out a positive idea into the universe, the universe will manifest it for our benefit and happiness. The ethical, moral, and spiritual motivations behind what a person projects with his or her thoughts is inconsequential. The so-called secret is that there is a "law of attraction" intrinsic to the human being and the universe, and if we learn to manipulate this law we can possess all those things that at one time were identified with the ideal American Dream. There are substantial faults with this notion. First, there is no new secret to this philosophy because it has been common sense in spiritual traditions since time immemorial. Second, there is nothing spiritual about this secret because it simply repackages a principle well known to depth psychologists and has nothing to do with higher spiritual ethics of compassion, kindness, and true wisdom. Finally, *The Secret* makes a fundamental error of ignoring the more essential spiritual need for making dramatic changes in people's lives, which can only be achieved by healthy motivation, commitment, discipline, and effort. Simply using our positive thoughts to attract a soulmate, a BMW, a new home, or better job will never instigate the necessary lifestyle changes people must make to live more enlightened and fulfilling lives.

What is most important for an investigation of boomer culture is not *The Secret*'s philosophy but why such a book and film have captured the imaginations of so many citizens and popular mass media, featured on *Oprah* and so many other shows.

In the 1970s, the Tibetan Buddhist teacher Chögyam Trungpa wrote a book, *Cutting Through Spiritual Materialism,* which was remarkably prophetic about the religious and spiritual landscape we are now experiencing during the twenty-first century. Trungpa's basic criticism of the way Westerners approach spirituality is that they refuse to let go of their ego-clinging when trying to develop themselves psychologically and spiritually. They meditate with an egoic intention such as "I gotta get there. I gotta get there," but the "I" is only the ego jabbering, and the ego is only an impermanent conditioned entity without any independent existence. While we might imagine that the ego can achieve happiness and peace, it in fact shuts us off from ultimately reaching a place that is essential and real. Once we realize that we are guided by our higher selves, our insights will change. We realize that nothing is permanent. Material things come and go because life is fluid. The trouble has been that almost all of today's postmodern belief systems would have us believe in permanency. In truth, everything, including our egos, changes all the time.

Today's pseudo-spirituality that is confined to the gratification of the ego—whether it be *The Secret* or the New Age movement in general—is an outgrowth of the boomers' need to find a quick fix, a spiritual bypass as it were, to avoid having to commit to the hard work of authentically transforming themselves. In my opinion it represents a desperate effort to find spiritual meaning in a society that has become overwhelmingly reductionist and denies the importance of vital spiritual values and the need to live by them to produce constructive, positive change.

Although the basic principle behind the "law of attraction" is valid, I would suggest raising it to a higher level. Instead of the Mercedes and more possessions that are impermanent, think of enduring universal qualities that you want to experience in your life. For example, if you focus on the quality of beauty, you will witness beauty where you never saw it before. You will even see beauty transpire through people who don't obviously exhibit beauty in their lives. If you think of solace and peace, you will feel quietude even when walking through the hustle of a large metropolis. If you think happy and pleasant thoughts you will discover yourself smiling at people you never smiled at before and chances are you will be rewarded with a smile in return. These are universal attributes that make our lives precious and full of excitement.

While conventional religion, particularly the kind of conservative evangelicalism that continues to increase in popularity, and New Age spirituality might appear to be diametrically opposed, I want to suggest they are more closely aligned than one might think; in fact they are two sides of the same coin. In the forms they appear to us now, both are boomer developments, although each can trace its roots to earlier generations' religious and spiritual experiences.

A major characteristic of a materialist culture is subjugation and acquisition. Conquest has in fact been a defining historical trait of Western civilization—colonialism, feudalism, Manifest Destiny's acquisition of territories, religious crusades to gain converts, male domination, and so on. The developed nations' embrace of globalization and free-market economics have been perceived by some scholars as a postmodern expression of colonialism. The primary goal, whether it be intentional or not, is to subjugate the national interests of poorer nations for the purpose of acquiring these nations' resources; the result is better profit margins for multinational corporations and developed governments. Media and corporate advertising, the pushing of drugs on television by the pharmaceutical industry, the news distortions of media's politically motivated spin doctors, can all be seen as extensions of colonialism. However, it is a colonialism far more subtle than what we have seen in the past; it concerns the colonization of the mind. This is a colonialism that subjugates the best of our mental capacities in order to gain our emotional support or get us to buy a particular product.

Both the religious materialism of conservative religion and the spiritual materialism of New Age thought are based upon the principles of subjugation and acquisition. The difference is that New Age beliefs operate at the individual level, whereas moralistic religion focuses on the collective level. The New Age reinforces the ego's self-gratification by promulgating a belief that a person can subjugate the universe for one's personal desires and wants. In this sense it is a distorted expression of the boomers' free-spirited revolt in favor of people manifesting their unique individuality in the 1960s and 1970s.

Conservative religion, on the other hand, does not promote the individuality of its believers. It is concerned with subjugating a large collective of people in order to acquire influence and power for furthering its moral agenda and belief system in society and the body politic. Unlike the New Age, the conservative religion of boomers does not trace its roots to the freethinking and self-exploration of the 1960s; instead it is a distortion of the Greatest Generation's community-based ethics that boomers grew up with.

Neither the New Age movement nor conservative religion is an answer for the critical social and spiritual needs of the twenty-first century. Although each has likely brought a degree of personal satisfaction to its adherents and has probably soothed anxieties and insecurities, neither can ever truly be a force for authentic spiritual change, either in individuals or a collective, because both are distortions of universal values shared by people all over the world. What is most needed today is an enlightened reinvention of positive values from the boomers' upbringing, and synergizing these with their rebellious spirit of idealism and life-affirming imagination. This is the boomer renewal I envision that is most needed to transform society for the benefit of future generations of young people whose world will be drastically different than the one we are living in today.

Living consciously means living spiritually. And living spiritually means paying attention to people in need. Most of us consider ourselves to be fine people, but our actions prove otherwise. One of the largest obstacles to breaking free of the chains preventing us from acting spiritually is our selfishness.

On a global scale, selfishness is manifested as multinational corporations and governments exploiting every inch of the planet. In Africa and Asia, massive poverty exists in part due to corporate intervention. Yet do we see Fortune 500 companies giving even a small portion of their revenues back to provide proper wells for clean drinking water? Do they invest in planting trees where they have devastated the environment through deforestation? Are they building medical facilities so local residents can combat local diseases such as malaria, dysentery, and tuberculosis? In almost all cases, there is little to no effort.

The heads of the multinational corporations are respected individuals. Most are religious people who donate large sums to their churches and synagogues. Almost every one of our politicians in Washington claims some form of religious belief or affiliation, and while they may hold sincere and legitimate belief in their faiths, their actions in the public sphere rarely demonstrate that they are truly spiritual or authentically compassionate. True decency involves helping other human beings, and attempting to improve the lives of those who have been wronged.

Swami Muktananda, a Hindu wise man from India, once said, "Expect nothing, and you will never be disappointed." The problem is, people generally expect more. They expect to receive in proportion to what they give, and that is not always what happens. As an example, you may have the consciousness that allows for compassion; you may be able to listen to others and understand them, but that doesn't mean that those others will have the same capacity to offer compassion in return. You can't expect another person to be just like you. So don't blame others if they're unable to give you what you've given them. If you have to give 90 percent in order to receive 10 percent, that's still a balanced equation if that's all the other person can give you in return. They gave what they could; that's their ability level. It's rare that you'll find someone who is able to give equally. Accept that, and you will truly be compassionate and caring.

Beginning with the reign of the Catholic Church when it became the worldly power over Europe, material power—the power to govern and control—replaced spiritual power. In the twenty-first century we are witnessing our world, nation, and social fabric dying. It is not simply dying from competitive greed and the exploitation and destruction of the environment. In a deeper way, it is also expiring from people's denial of a spirit that authentically connects and unifies us all. Our society will never be healed by corporate executives, new scientific advances, and politicians. Both the New Age movement and the pervasive conservative religions that dominate American religiosity are blinded by their spiritual materialism, thereby fundamentally denying the dynamics of an authentic spirituality.

These movements are trying to heal what doesn't need healing—because our true and genuine spiritual selves are already whole and pure. The authentic self can only be found by developing our inner life; it is the only trustworthy leader capable of expressing the wisdom that can guide and heal ourselves and others.

Happiness

There are several factors that contribute to our development from childhood into adulthood and will ultimately determine how well we will fulfill our individual purpose in life. Two of these factors are most important and frequently play a tug-of-war with each other. One is our individual energy, a birthright that we are born with when we emerge into this world. It includes all of a child's latent talents and skills that, if nurtured conscientiously, will allow the child to blossom and live a productive and healthy life. The other, which is more important for this discussion, is the conditioning we absorb from our environment, which includes our parents and family members, our school and our culture. This includes not only the verbal lessons that children are given and the actions they witness, but also the energy, positive and negative, that they absorb from their environment. For this reason it is not unusual to see a frantic child accompanied by a frantic parent.

Last year I had a conversation with Professor Tal Ben-Shahar, a Harvard professor of positive psychology whose courses in happiness are the most popular on Harvard's campus. Professor Ben-Shahar estimates that 94 percent of all college students in America today are overly stressed and unhappy at their core. If true, and I believe he is correct, this is a frightening statistic. Young people today have been conditioned by the pressures of their boomer parents and by the onslaught of mass media and advertising to achieve a vision of success that is nothing more than giving obeisance to the deities of wealth and possessions. Moreover, they are taught that only aggressive competition, combined with distrust toward anyone other than oneself, is the means for reaching this goal. In the twenty-first century, happiness is sorely limited to whether you have more than your neighbor.

However, if we consider the statistic that only 6 percent of young adults today are authentically happy, that means that almost our entire society, nearly everyone who interacts with a growing kid, is also fundamentally unhappy. This is a strong indictment against the world boomers have created for themselves and their children. Is it any wonder then that our leaders—in government, corporations, educational systems, and faith communities—ignore the important issues for improving the essential quality of the citizens' lives that they represent? Our entire media world of talking heads is mostly populated by unhappy, disgruntled individuals.

There is an insightful saying of the Buddha, "Thousands of candles can be lighted from a single candle, and the life of the candle will not be shortened. Happiness never decreases by being shared." But the Buddha is speaking about a happiness only found in a place of contentment within ourselves. Buddha's only possessions were his robes and begging bowl. All the possessions we own— including all the speculative assets boomers have assumed are theirs for the taking—are subject to change and decay. Imagine the stress and fear of all the families who are losing their homes from fore- closures, watching their investments and possessions decrease during the recession that commenced in late 2007. There are so many people in America today who are desperately unhappy because they have not acquired the American Dream promised them. Particularly in this worsening economy, financial hardship is an ongoing concern. But the more we focus exclusively on material issues, the longer we will overlook the pervasive, epidemic problem of people defining the value of their lives in terms of reaching a particular social status and the amount of possessions they can surround themselves with.

It may come as a shock to some boomer readers to learn that on February 19, 2008, the *New York Times* reported that the Centers for Disease Control noted a sharp 20 percent increase in suicides among middle-aged baby boomers (between the ages of forty-five and fifty-four) over a five-year period. The rate among boomer women rose 31 percent. At a mundane level, I believe our society's overuse and abuse of antidepressant drugs is largely a triggering factor behind this statistic. More importantly, however, are the causes for why so many boomers have a need to take antidepressants.

There is a deeper and more spiritually based rationale for the rise in suicides among boomers, male and female alike. I recall a conversation I had with Sandra Ingerman, a psychologist and an accomplished shaman in New Mexico. She stated the problem well, "If we don't want to live, the universe will create the conditions to shorten our lives." This is a very powerful statement and food for thought.

Boomer men's emotional immaturity and insecurity about their aging and loss of sexual vitality has partially contributed to the depressed social climate many middle-aged women are forced to live with. Being too preoccupied with themselves and their careers, boomer men retreat from their inner world where life is sensual, and instead chase after the youth that is receding away from them. Finding a woman many years their junior to try to re-create their earlier sense of sexual vitality is an escape from and denial of aging. As a result many boomer women have been feeling the loss of male companionship and intimacy.

For boomer children, possessions weren't generally viewed as permanent but were to be explored, experienced, and then let go. Your joy was in using and sharing more than in owning. Once we became adults, though, we didn't want anyone else to touch our things. One floor is only for the president, the executive vice president, and the executive secretary. Everyone else is kept out. But the president, the executive vice president, and the executive secretary may not know who they really are. They may get their identities from their titles, and from the fact that they have their own floor.

What happens when you cease to base your identity on what you possess? You find other things more meaningful, such as a sunset, the sound of ocean waves, or the graceful movement of an animal. You're freer to experiment with new jobs, new activities, new environments for living, new people. I truly believe that unless you are able to separate yourself from your possessions, you will never find true happiness or see the beauty in this world.

Something I have noticed during my meetings with parents and their children, with few exceptions, is that the children of boomer parents who have continued to live in the spirit of the ideals that earlier defined their generation—dedication to practicing some form of viable spirituality and realizing that the quality of life is more essential than the quantity of things they can consume—are happier, more content, and more balanced. On the other hand, those parents whose lives are overwhelmed with work, preoccupied with keeping a career schedule that doesn't permit quality time with their children, and who are constantly competing with the Joneses, have the most unhappy children. Their children are also among those with the most learning difficulties such as ADD and ADHD.

You have probably heard of AA and OA, Alcoholics Anonymous and Overeaters Anonymous. But if you ask me, we could really use an additional self-help organization: TAA: Thing Addicts Anonymous. Millions of baby boomers need to join such a group. They're thing addicts.

Now don't get me wrong, I think the boomer generation is wonderful in many ways and they've accomplished much. They freed us from many stagnant notions of age-appropriate behavior, sex-appropriate roles, and codes of dress. As a consequence, people are a lot freer to be who they want to be than they were several decades ago. In the area of parenting, boomers advocated to include fathers in the experience of childbirth and in the daily care of young children. In the field of health, they're largely responsible for introducing more natural healing modalities. People condemn this generation for being pleasure-seeking, but I think pleasure-seeking has certain benefits, and Americans should be experiencing more of the pleasures in life that contribute to our happiness. But that pleasure-seeking has to be experience-seeking, not thing-seeking, and boomers often confuse the two.

This confusion may have to do with the era in which baby boomers grew up—their parents lived through World War II and all the deprivation and shortages that went with it. After the war, they felt they deserved a few pleasures, one of which was having a family; hence the baby boom itself. But people were also able to indulge in a variety of new possessions, such as houses, appliances, and cars, all of which went along with the new suburban way of life that many Americans were then adopting. A good economy, the growth of our highway system, and the development of cheap mass-building techniques were all factors contributing to the rapid growth of suburbs after the war. People's sense of optimism and entitlement impelled them to start experiencing the good life. We had won the war, after all; America was the greatest country on earth, and there was no reason we shouldn't live like it. Children who grew up in the late 1940s, 1950s, and early 1960s were surrounded by these good feelings, and with the idea that material acquisitions were part and parcel of being an American in the middle of the twentieth century.

During the Cold War with the Soviet Union, it was almost as if buying things was a patriotic act, because doing so demonstrated how well our system worked. We still witness vestiges of this thinking today with America's dwindling economy in the twenty-first century. Repeatedly we hear politicians and economists speaking about ways to spur the economy by legislating changes that will increase consumer spending. For the listener, one would think that the entire value of the nation is based upon how much citizens can spend and consume. The sad fact is that our leaders also equate the happiness of the nation with citizens' capacity to purchase more and more stuff.

Another factor facilitating the acquisition of things was the development of plastics. One of the reasons baby boomer children were able to have more toys than the previous generation did was that plastic was beginning to supplant metal and wood as a cheaper material for toy manufacture. In addition, as toys became cheaper and Americans richer, families could afford to toss toys out and get new ones in a way they never could before. Hence we started to become a "throw-away culture" in the 1950s. Today people are tossing away computers like they did used toys, after a year or two of use.

But there is good news today, and it's that some of the baby boomers and other age groups are asking themselves the question: Why has a "standard of living" always been equated with how much stuff you own? And they are concluding that possessions are not necessarily the most important part of the good life. There's a burgeoning trend called "voluntary simplicity." This involves cutting down on what one has in terms of things while increasing activities that bring a sense of joy and happiness, such as spending more time with family and friends, participating in local activities that support community values, and enjoying the pleasures of nature and hobbies such as gardening and hiking.

There is an interesting contemporary lesson about happiness to be learned from the other side of the globe. The king of the small Buddhist Himalayan kingdom of Bhutan, in defiance of the large international and multilateral agencies' attempts to judge the value his nation based on productivity and wealth, trashed the idea of a Gross National Product (GNP) as a realistic factor for determining Bhutan's health. Instead, King Jigme Wangchuck promoted the idea that a nation's health should be determined by the degree of happiness experienced in its population. Hence he coined the term "Gross National Happiness" because the joy and peace one experiences in the presence of the Bhutanese, which is almost unmatched by any other people around the world—except for perhaps isolated indigenous peoples—is a result of material and spiritual development occurring side by side. For the Bhutanese, "voluntary simplicity" is simply a way of life that has existed for centuries. But chances are a government agency devoted to assuring the happiness of American citizens wouldn't work, because voluntary simplicity is an individual effort that requires people to understand the benefits to be gained by unraveling the clutter from their lives.

The reasons people turn toward voluntary simplicity are several. First, many people are simplifying their lives to save money; they can no longer afford the upper-middle-class suburban lifestyle that is still put forth as the American ideal. Second, there's the environmental concern, with many advocates of voluntary simplicity feeling that America's high-living, throw-away lifestyle puts a huge drain on the planet and is unfair to less-developed countries and to future generations as well. Also, modern American life has become so complex and demanding that people get tense trying to fit everything they're supposed to do into a twenty-four-hour day; thus, it makes sense to try to simplify the demands and cut down on stress. Further, some are drawn to this movement for philosophical and spiritual reasons; for example, they permit themselves frequent quiet time to rejuvenate their inner happiness and peace. This in turn helps them to speak, act, and share in the most harmonious and constructive ways with their children and others.

We work toward making our lives comfortable. Comforts provide a sense of security. But they also prevent us from trying anything new. We become afraid to quit our jobs and find new work, change relationships, or even change the way we eat, dress, or comb our hair. New situations create discomfort. We have no way of predicting how we are going to feel and what is going to happen to us. Comfort also creates complacency. Complacency stops the growth process. It prevents us from asking questions that are critical to growth and improvement.

When people stop taking risks, they stagnate. Joy is no longer there, and they don't see the happy side of life. They are only bitter and cynical. Why? Because the only perspective they have is of the ferment that is occurring around them. Who creates that ferment? They do. But who are they going to blame? Everybody else, or they blame circumstances.

When you are willing to act differently and take some risks, before long you will begin to feel comfortable doing something else differently. Soon you will start looking forward to experiencing life and not being afraid. Suddenly, your tiny view of life expands and your life is all the richer for it.

The happy person is balanced. And balanced people appreciate what they have. This is one of the most important things I have learned about life, and why I insist: Stop always thinking that there's someone or something missing from your life and that you won't be happy until you find it. And if you think that someone out there has the answer—the Dalai Lama, Wayne Dyer, Deepak Chopra, or Gary Null—you're wrong. We don't have the answers for you. The best we can do is offer some questions and guidance.

Once you know what you don't want in life, you have to determine what you do want—not in terms of possessions, but in terms of meaning. You must create your meaning. Start to picture who you want to be and how you want to live. If you don't do that, it will never happen. There is a marvelous saying, "The pull of the future is greater than the push of the past." When we focus on the past, paying too much attention to our old self and the traumas and upsets that condition our thinking, and permit that to be the shaper and guider of our lives, we are pushed along to and fro. Consequently, we lose all sense of control over where we are going. On the other hand, if we allow ourselves to be in the moment, surrendering our past in order to be open to the future, then we are pulled effortlessly toward the opportunities that will improve and transform us. It is this second way that enables us to cast off the dross from our being to reveal our new self.

Finally, make the commitment to be unpredictable. When you do that you will begin to unfurl the person you truly are. Doing so provides us with an exhilarating sense of freedom, as if the chains holding us to past conditions were sliding away from our limbs. You must have the confidence to re-create experiences of pleasure or peace of mind every day. Remember that the authentic self finds happiness and a sense of peace in life, and that you're entitled to them.

Neglecting the Power of Silence

I remember an occasion when a communication satellite malfunctioned, knocking out service to many of the nation's paging devices for a couple of days. This technological breakdown was serious enough that it made front-page news. But the really interesting thing was that many pager owners weren't all that upset. In fact, they were quite relieved. With their beepers temporarily silenced, there was one less bit of noise infiltrating their lives and demanding a prompt response. For a short while, their world became a little quieter, a little calmer.

This led me to imagine a scenario: What if all our nonessential communications could go on the fritz for awhile? Emergency services would still be in place, but otherwise there would be no telephones, faxes, TV, radio, or e-mail. The effect would be like that of the satellite breakdown ten times over: People's lives would be much quieter, and the subtle sounds of nature would come to the fore. People would be able to think more clearly. They'd have more time to examine the meaning of their lives, instead of just scrambling to keep up with the trappings. In short, they would discover the power of silence.

This kind of selective power outage probably won't happen. But on an individual level we can make it happen to some extent, simply by turning off the appropriate switches when we can. There's another simple step we can take—we can stop talking so much. Then we can sit back, or go for a walk in the open air, and revel in the quiet.

Members of the baby boom generation are sorely in need of silence, because many have been silence-deprived all their lives. This is the first television generation. In addition to television, this generation was the first to grow up with telephones as a birthright, not as an option. The number of automobiles in the United States boomed along with the number of babies in the 1950s and 1960s, bringing increased traffic, noise, and destruction of natural environments. There is even "light noise"—unless you live in a rural area—which prevents people from ever being able to see the full beauty of the starry sky. Excessive noise, light interference, and the increase of electromagnetic waves from computers, cell phones, and household appliances all have a profound physiological effect on a person's quality of sleep.

Professor Rubin Naiman, a sleep researcher at the University of Arizona's Program in Integrative Medicine has studied "night blindness," which is the effect on a person's health and psychology of being deprived of darkness and bombarded by emissions from electronic devices and excessive light stimulation. According to Naiman, sleep disorders are epidemic today and affect all generations alike.

During the past year, Science News Daily—a leading reporting service for the most recent scientific research literature—has been noting a large increase in studies that show poor and deficient sleep in all age groups as contributing to disorders such as impaired mental function, obesity, diabetes, childhood learning difficulties, and more. Yet this is simply a continuum and increase of the beginnings of a noise culture inherited by the boomers. Add up all these factors and you can see why silence is something that many of today's adults did not grow up with but so desperately need.

A woman came down to my holistic retreat to attend a series of workshops, but she and a small group of people talked nonstop. There was no introspection. I kept telling them that their best time would be spent in silence, doing nothing except being with nature. No one listened. The woman wasn't going to stay a second week until I sat her down and told her that she had not learned anything because the most important message is always the silent one. I asked her to spend a second week there in silence, and she did.

During the second week, I asked every guest to eat in silence. I provided candlelight and flower arrangements. There was no conversation. For the first time, people knew what it was to eat in an environment conducive to inner tranquility. Now they were aware of what they were eating. They lost weight. They felt energized. Later when I took them out to sit quietly and listen to the wind, they suddenly could hear a symphony in the wind. They could allow every distracting thought to leave their minds.

People would tell me, marveling, that they could hear a thousand different sounds in the wind. "I heard the top of the palm trees moving. And I heard the grass moving. I heard the animals in the background, and the birds." All the sounds had been there before, but everyone had tuned them out because they were focused on their own chatter.

When we can finally break through to place our energy in the moment of silence, we are able to transcend the normal boundaries of visual perception, smell, and taste. We become integrated. Like a bird, which never contemplates its death while flying, we don't experience fear of falling from the sky. But most us fly with fear.

It's interesting how an experience can change so completely when it is encountered with integrated thoughts. I could have you sit down for an hour to meditate, and you might wonder about whether your children are all right and where your husband is. If your mind is somewhere else, you are not integrated. On the other hand, you could be there in the moment. That's where healing occurs.

Only by being alone can you experience a silent mind that allows you to think about who you are, not who you've been told you are, or who you should be. Then no relationship will ever take precedence over your self. We have the mistaken notion in our society that the high point of our adult life is a relationship. I find that for most people that's very unhealthy. It's normal and human to relate to people and to share with them, but you should never be your relationship. Because what happens is that you cannot differentiate your self from the relationship. You never have a sense of being a complete and whole person. You're always attached at the psyche to someone else. And then you get caught up in power struggles. When you tie yourself up in knots trying to find your self-worth in another person there can never be any authentic interior space that's truly your own.

When we learn to be present with ourselves in silence and begin to learn the lessons of silence, we begin to observe how our mind and feelings function. You might ask yourself, what comes first, the thought or the emotion? The thought always arrives first. A thought is a word or a sentence or an entire idea that you've created. Consider how many times you've thought about something that you didn't do and should have done, or that you did and wished you hadn't. How many opportunities have you had and lost, and then relived a thousand times in your mind? Every time you relive a moment, you relive it by creating thoughts.

The thought, then, is not the reality. But how many times have you made thoughts real? For instance, we're in a small Southern town. There's an all-white audience. Suddenly, a black person comes in and sits down. How many people are going to think a negative, fearful, racist thought and make it seem as if it's real?

Thoughts are not real. They're merely constructs. No one can have only positive thoughts. Even if you meditate, not all of the thoughts that arise from the surface of the mind will be positive. And the negative thoughts are often followed by an emotion of fear, anxiety, insecurity, resentment, or anger. You might decide that meditation, or yoga, or correct breathing isn't the only antidote to make you relieve your stress, so you look to health food, vitamins, or juices to improve the quality of your health. But these aren't going to change your life in any essential way; rather, it's your attitude that is going to change your life. Your life's only going to change after you learn to curb your criticism toward yourself and others.

There is nothing more damaging than an overly critical mind. If you need to do everything right you may experience some failure along the way. Then you're going to beat up on yourself. So we need to be comfortable in silence and use that silence to focus only on actualizing what is constructive. Think in terms of watching your thoughts parade in front of you and saying, No ... not that one ... yes, that one I like. That one supports my intentions. That's healthy. I'll take it in. Just let go of everything else because it's not constructive. This is an excellent way to get out of our destructive patterns and to find solutions to our problems.

Universal Outrage

Not long ago I produced a documentary about cancer and the vested corporate and medical interests involved with this disease. During the program, I provided a forum for many viewers to speak. Many patients felt various kinds of anger and outrage. When we use terms like anger, rage, and outrage, we need to be careful about what each refers to. Anger can sometimes be a positive emotion in that it is an expression of energy. But realize that there is a difference between anger and rage. Rage can hurt; anger can create change. In fact, I can't understand people who never feel angry. It seems to me that if you don't get angry at things, you have no passion for life. Anger most often has a very personalized quality. For example, if someone betrays me in some way, I might feel anger toward that person. Rage is when my anger takes complete possession of me whereby I lose reason and seek retaliation.

Then there is what I consider to be a higher form of anger, which we can call outrage. Outrage is not personal. I believe it is an inherent attribute of life that is expressed when something of great injustice is done that betrays the spirit of human reason and universal laws. For example, if I am watching the news and witness footage of a genocide in Africa or a story about a corporation knowingly destroying the environment and people's lives, I feel outrage. My own person is not being targeted by the genocide or the corporation, nevertheless I experience these actions as a violation of universal decency and the dignity of human life. Most of my documentaries are the products of an outrage I have felt toward how the medical establishment and other vested corporate and government interests have abused their power and resources, injuring and even destroying the lives of innocent citizens. There is a segment in my film *Gulf War Syndrome: Killing Our Own* in which I show pictures of Iraqi children who died as a result of the first bombing, suffering from poisoning by the bombs' depleted uranium and from the subsequent sanctions that prohibited Iraq from receiving medicine and equipment to assure functioning water facilities and civil infrastructures. The photos show innocent children inflicted with a wide range of birth deformities, previously unobserved cancers, and rare diseases due to toxic chemical exposure. Many people who have seen the film told me they cried while viewing this segment and felt an over-whelming sense of outrage toward our government's decision to attack Iraq. That is what outrage does. It opens our heart toward another person who has been violated indiscriminately and against all reason, and instills in us a desire to act to correct the wrong.

Most people get so comfortable and secure in their predictable lives that there is no anger and outrage left to project as a positive emotion. Remember the outrage of some of the baby boom genera-tion as they protested the Vietnam War? Where has that motivation to actualize feelings of outrage gone? When outrage is actualized positively, it can be a powerful, constructive force for correcting the wrongs in the world. It was this kind of outrage that motivated Ralph Nader to go to Washington to protect American citizens from a wide range of abuses and that attracted young idealists and well-educated lawyers and activists from New England to create Nader's Raiders. It is a shame that boomers have forgotten how to feel out-rage and instead have resigned themselves to the apathy of living self-centered lives. Today we are in urgent need of more outrage from aging boomers in order to jump-start new constructive and enlightened activism to improve our society.

Children of the Boomers

Occasionally on my radio broadcasts I have guests from the younger generation—the children of boomers—who have published impor-tant books or who have taken on the mantle of being spokespersons for their generation. I also have opportunities to speak with the young people who work in our offices and I ask them for their opin-ions about their parents and the boomer generation. Although most of them admire and have been influenced by much of what boomers produced during the 1960s and 1970s, my impression is that the overall sentiment toward their parents' generation is one of disgust.

Kids whose parents continue to hold the higher ideals representing the best of the boomers' past, who walk their talk, show a greater appreciation for their parents than those whose parents have lost themselves in the superficiality of American mass media and the endless pursuit of possessions, money, and quick-fix schemes to try to feel more secure about themselves. One of the more common criticisms I hear when I ask young adults about what they dislike most in their parents' generation is their obsession with consumerism, their careers, and superficial interests.

For example, not long ago I read an e-mail from a well-educated young man in his early thirties who grew up in a family that was very influential and popular in pioneering the burst of exploration into Eastern mysticism during the 1960s. He summarized very succinctly how many of the boomers' children look upon their parents' generation today:

> Some of us have a deep respect for the baby boomer generation and the earlier culture it produced. In particular we are impressed with their music, their progressive politics—especially the civil rights movement—their proud, unapologetic identification with spirituality and a certain frank, unembarrassed emotional expression. In some cases we see their early example as something we would like to replicate in our own generation. However, there is a feeling that the baby boomers, after innovating many projects and advancements, have lost their edge. They have become more passive and less discriminating. For example, the generation who challenged the assumptions of conventional religion now seems to passively accept the assumptions and dogmas of New Age and fundamentalist religions. There is an embarrassing indiscriminateness in that generation's hopping on the bandwagon

of New Age crazes in health and spirituality, which seem to me to be shallow and uninteresting commodifications of the impulse to explore, which earlier defined this group's visionary and expansive spiritual evolution. Their current lack of discrimination and acceptance of mass media versions of music, entertainment, politics, social values, and spirituality unfortunately makes me doubt they are a group worth much consideration anymore.

I believe that underlying this young man's sentiments is a larger perception that the boomers are alienated from themselves, their children, parents, communities, and just about everything else that is vital and imaginative for experiencing life's fullness. In many cases, young people feel a resentment toward the boomer generation for producing a society filled with strip malls and an insane ethic that everything should be exploited for personal short-term gain. Or else young adults are too numb to notice or feel there is anything authentic and real around them. This has been the primary conditioning they received from their boomer families, education, and environment, and so in some ways it is all they really know.

While preparing for the publication of this book, I had a conversation with Pir Zia Inayat-Khan, one of the few authentic spiritual teachers to have arisen from the present younger generation. When asked about his perceptions concerning his generation's lack of spiritual ideals and their complacency toward civic activism, he agreed that this was largely the case for the vast majority of young adults today. They entertain a wild menagerie of eclectic ideas lacking any focused direction and are adrift in a sea of information, consumerism, and competition, which seems to follow the mantra that "life is uncertain so reap and enjoy all you can." Speaking about his own education while growing up outside San Francisco, Pir Zia said he was utterly bored and found no inspiration in what and how he was being taught. In fact, he fell into serious doubt that he would ever make anything of himself in life. This is not an uncommon experience among young adults regarding their education during their growing years. The further degradation of American education to a level of banal mediocrity is another contribution boomers can be thanked for.

Partially to blame is their boomer parents' information-based culture, which has overwhelmed young adults' minds with nonessential data that offers little for living a happy and rewarding life. Any boomer who experimented with hallucinogenic drugs during the adventuresome 1960s and 1970s will remember the overload of thoughts and images pummeling their minds. This is an accurate analogy for what our obsession with information has done to the minds of young adults. Boomers have built for themselves a vast hallucination. The problem with a hallucination is that you experience it alone. There is no one sharing the images and thoughts crowding in upon you. Likewise, we are so busy in our hallucination of consumerism and career-oriented success in order to fill the void left by insecurities and fears that we are unaware of how isolated we have become. There is less of a vital lifeline connecting us with our elders, our children, our friends, and communities.

The boomers' experiment with building a social hallucination populated with mental and physical stimuli blasting across everyone's senses is part of this generation's legacy to its children. Little wonder that boomers might see their children as if walking through a dream, indulging themselves in the immediate, short-term pleasures society offers them. What else is a hallucination except a play of the mind?

Another fundamental difficulty young adults face is detaching themselves from the culture of entitlement they were raised in. In the meritocracy of the Greatest Generation, discipline, focus, study, and mastery would result in the gradual achievement of rewards for a person's efforts. Learning mastery is a gradual process. Accomplishing small feats generates confidence and a sense of satisfaction to undertake greater deeds. For better or worse, it was the boomers' conditioning in mastery through accomplishment that expanded Wall Street and built huge megacomplexes such as Silicon Valley. Boomers also launched great advancements in science and technology at a rate unprecedented in human history.

When boomers replaced merit with entitlement, they were essentially saying to their children, "You don't have to prove anything to us because you are already deserving of being rewarded simply because you are here." Over the years of running an office with anywhere between thirty and one hundred people at a given time, I have had ample opportunities to closely observe the work ethic of young adults. I frequently witness the detrimental effects of entitlement on these young adult minds in their attitude and relationship to work. Often they demand to work on their own terms. Their loyalty to what they accomplish only lasts until something paying a higher salary comes along.

At the same, I also observe great potential for young adults on the horizon. They have keen, visionary qualities awaiting to be actualized. Although some boomers who are the dynamic leaders in America are unlikely to step down after reaching retirement age, young people today are starting to realize they can exert positive change on a grassroots civic level thanks to their natural affinity for the Internet and other high-tech communication. If they can discover themselves as more deeply connected with others at a spiritual level, latent ideals will come to the fore, and they can constructively use their unique technical and problem-solving skills to initiate positive change.

The Boomers' Legacy

Everyone is ultimately disposable. That's the way life on this planet works. People don't like the idea of being impermanent, but no matter how important they are, every person and every thing in life is transitory. Everyone who ever lived was disposable. As important as Buddha or Christ were, they were impermanent too. They helped humankind, they gave people new insights, but ultimately they came and went. It's what they left afterwards that people remember and treasure.

We remember those who live honestly and who earnestly seek to create beauty. We love the honesty of expression in music, literature, poetry, and art. We also cherish people's contributions made on a more personal level to improve the lives of their families and friends and to enrich their communities.

The sad fact of the matter is that the baby boomer generation has left a legacy for future generations that is fundamentally unsustainable and impermanent. When boomers were handed the baton from the Greatest Generation to further shape the country, they ended up placing their trust in the very things that brought unhappiness and disease. All those things and values they thought would bring them happiness, such as the perfect spouse, the perfect job, and piles of possessions, led in so many cases to disheartenment. When boomers reached their ascendancy during the late 1980s and onwards, they dismantled many of the institutions and infrastructures that were the gifts of the Greatest Generation's legacy: Family and community cohesion and togetherness eroded and were replaced by the highest divorce rates and single-parent families in American history; the tradition of feeling assured that there was a job for you disappeared when downsizing and corporate mergers based on the whims of those who stood to gain the most wealth became the norm; those boomers who came into corporations and institutions as trust babies, never having needed to prove they were worthy of their inheritance through hard work and effort, virtually destroyed what was handed to them; and the appreciation of spending within one's means was replaced by a culture of debt and speculation that now contributes to America's uncertain economic future and its standing in the community of nations. Perhaps worse, the boomer values of consumption and exploitation—corporate and individual—coupled with its addiction to wastefulness continue to deplete the nation's environmental resources at an unprecedented rate.

The parents of boomers appreciated and honored the inevitability of approaching death. For this reason, leaving a legacy to their children was an important statement affirming their lives' worth and purpose. Many others performed good deeds in their communities and died with the comfort of knowing that they would be remembered for their kindness. Innovators who built businesses and companies saw them as a permanent legacy that they envisioned would continue to thrive for generations to come. Of course, communications professor Leonard Steinhorn at American University does note that polls taken in the mid-1990s reveal that most Greatest Generation senior citizens still oppose interracial marriage, divorce, the rise of working mothers, and gay rights, in addition to insisting that young people should follow the dictates of their elders. But while many of their beliefs, allegiances, and convictions may seem out of touch today, the Greatest Generation's intentions were genuine.

The United Nations' official definition of sustainability can be paraphrased as: to develop and use natural resources in a responsible and ethical manner that does not deprive future generations from providing for their own needs while relying upon those same resources. As I mentioned above, the boomer legacy includes indiscriminate abuse of the environment. For example, today's monopolistic agro-industry, which has ruined the legacy of the family farm, is completely nonsustainable for long-term food production. As geomorphologist Professor David Montgomery at the University of Washington told me, the earth's topsoil is more fragile than the top layer of the human skin. All of the world's agricultural production is based on the couple feet of topsoil beneath our feet. When that is depleted, the land turns barren. This is only one example of megacorporations' misuse of natural resources. The same is true for water, the quality of plant foods due to genetic engineering, forests, and more. Former World Bank vice president Ismail Serageldin predicted that the wars of this century will increase and will focus primarily over water access and rights. Today more than five million people, mostly children, die annually from impure drinking water. Americans across all generations seem to maintain the insulated belief that such problems will never happen here.

Every boomer should ask him- or herself, *Will the legacy of my generation assure the well-being and healthy lives of our children?* My own answer is a definitive *no*. This is what I call the "boomer dilemma." How then do boomers restore their legacy, which is now nothing more than a broken-down palace?

To the United Nations' definition of sustainability above, I would also add human sustainability and spiritual sustainability. Human sustainability refers to restoring universal values to our lifestyles, our institutions, our communities, and families. Making this happen requires a dramatic shift from the current perception of boomers as a "Me" generation to becoming an "Us" generation that respects our society's diversity and pluralism, whether it be race, gender, religious orientation, political allegiance, or social status. In order to make a society's health sustainable, citizens must shift their perspective away from themselves and toward the well-being of others. Spiritual sustainability refers to developing our inner life and mindfulness. Our attention toward improving our personal lives, learning to become mindful of the consequences of our choices, and discovering happiness and peace within ourselves are prior conditions for any viable and sustainable act we might initiate to improve society's human sustainability.

Pioneering a new path, or restoring a path forgotten and ignored, is not easy. But we can still live vibrant lives and accomplish great deeds, large or small. We can take on new, more awakened roles in our families, our communities, and local organizations. But we have to make concerted choices about caring for our inner life if these things are going to happen.

We can begin this process by first focusing our attention upon universal values—beauty, kindness, compassion, joy, and excitement, and on the inherent energy within ourselves to accomplish noble deeds. During our spare moments, rather than giving heed to things that are impermanent, we can instead focus on a universal value within ourselves. Whenever you find the urge to buy more things or to replace something that is still perfectly functional with a new and improved model, stop to investigate your motivations. There is no need to continue our neurotic obsession with searching outside ourselves for answers. The more we seek for external solutions, the greater the personal angst we experience. Years ago when I was travelling by bus from West Virginia to New York, I remember it being hot and stuffy. They didn't have air conditioning on the buses, and it was a seventeen-hour ride. I remember a woman sitting so peacefully and calmly throughout it all that outside of Pittsburgh I asked her, "Aren't you uncomfortable?" She said, "No, I'm just thinking nice thoughts."

I thought, *I'm thinking about how uncomfortable I am. And this guy is smoking a smelly little cigar behind me.* And here was this woman. She taught me something important in the midst of an unpleasant experience. Her spirit touched me and strengthened me.

We should also frequently reflect on the impermanence of our lives. As Buddhists often like to say, the only thing we must do in life is die. From the moment of birth, all of life is simply a walkway leading to death. One of the problems with the paradigm of permanence is that you know in your heart it's not true. But you've already given your loyalty to that belief, hence you are living a conflicted existence, which creates a sense of emptiness. On the other hand, when you live in the moment and accept the moment as being impermanent, you don't feel betrayed and dying is no longer threatening.

Having seen what has happened to senior citizens of their parents' generation, boomers are kicking and screaming over the prospects of aging. Like everything else they struggle to possess and accumulate in their nests, clinging onto youthfulness is just another thing to possess. Retirement is an idea that not all boomers are happy with because it means they will be ushered into the world of their aging parents whom they have ignored or neglected. Therefore, boomers are fearful of handing over the baton to the younger generation.

I can't emphasize enough to boomers that so many young people in their twenties and thirties are disgusted with the legacy their parents are bequeathing them. They think, *Step aside and go to pasture. You had your chance. It is our turn to take over.* Yet for many aging boomers, especially those who have dynamic personalities and who have taken on leadership roles in the reshaping of the American landscape, this is like a call from the grim reaper. The boomers' response is, *Hold on. It is not our time to fade away into a misty fog of insignificance.*

At the same time, boomers are the first generation to believe they can actually defy aging. Because they are accustomed to success, boomers expect success in defeating the coming of old age. It is true that believing that it is necessary to age "on schedule" is perhaps one of the worst mistakes a person can make. Due to past conditioning, many boomers have a set of expectations about how people are supposed to look and behave during each decade of life. Today our knowledge about aging has expanded tremendously. Those who follow the older model they internalized years ago, say in the 1950s and 1960s, are going to shortchange themselves throughout life, and may actually be lessening the years and quality of their lives.

The average life expectancy in America has increased almost a decade during the past half-century (from sixty-eight in 1950 to seventy-eight in the twenty-first century). Boomers realize that they don't have to act or look old at any particular time. So today, we have senior citizens working past the traditional retirement age, some runners in their eighties completing marathons, and authors in their nineties writing books.

All the knowledge and information in the world is not going to be of any benefit if a person's attitude about life is negative. Boomers have exerted too much effort achieving and consuming at the expense of experiencing the wonders of the world around them. They have placed their enjoyment on hold in order to chase after some magical moment in the future when they will feel completely secure. Now they are starting to regret not having taken more time to nurture themselves and to develop meaningful relationships with others. People obsess about what they might have been and what they could have done. We need to surrender our delusions and regrets and live solely with what we are willing to be.

For both women and men of the baby boom generation the bottom line is this: If you're going to avoid the aging-on-schedule trap, first and foremost you're going to have to want to. You're going to have to feel good enough about yourself and your life to want to get out there and shine, for years to come. You're going to have to want to try new things and take on new tasks, develop new habits, and possibly make big changes.

If boomers are to consciously address the dilemma of their legacy, they need to create authentic meaning in their lives so that they are not forgotten after they leave. Then their lives will not really be disposable. The memory of what they have left will be honored. In that way they will live forever.

Who Do You Want to Be When You Grow Up?

Not too long ago a middle-aged woman came to my Florida ranch to work on our production projects. She had a pedigree background: a privileged family, a Vassar education, and a very lucrative career at a major Wall Street firm. I asked her why she gave up a prestigious career to come to a ranch and work a low-profile job. Her response defines the current state of American society and the polarization between the generations of boomer parents and their children.

> It was because everywhere I looked I saw hyper-stimulated and aggressive alpha males and females competing to get ahead—and for no ethical purpose other than the personal gratification of showing off who they are and what they own. Eventually I felt spiritually violated and I came to the realization that to save my soul I couldn't work in such an environment anymore.

Later she described the financial environment that now governs our economy. Financial institutions today are comprised of two groups: the baby boomers who created the dominant empires of unsustainable investment and the young turks—the "Wolves on Wall Street" as a recent book title calls them—who have no ethical and moral backbone to inspire them to act conscientiously. The entire system has bought the politicians and legislators in order to avoid any sensible regulation that would prevent them from capitalizing on the destructive effects of their speculative schemes. The rules of the game are simple: everyone and everything can be exploited for personal gain and social climbing. Or, as this woman described it to me, we now have "an orgy of excess." For example, none of our policy makers and leaders, who are steeped in strategic ties with lobbyists' vested interests, are realistically addressing the underlying causes for the subprime mortgage mess and the vast personal debts Americans face today.

People are succumbing to the slogans and promises of politicians, analysts, and the media as a rationale for speculating indiscriminately on their assets to get the larger home, the bigger car, the next vacation. For the boomers and young adults who have already achieved success, it is not a matter of raising themselves out of poverty, but instead of raising their contorted self-image to celebrity status.

There was a time in the 1960s and early 1970s when boomers offered the nation a new paradigm that was based upon more enlightened civic virtues. Even if a boomer was not a member of an activist organization, he or she more than likely respected those who voiced the ideals for societal renewal. This is why we still remember the names of Rachel Carson, Cesar Chavez, Daniel and Philip Berrigan, Eldridge Cleaver, and Ralph Nader. What differentiates the boomer generation of yesterday from the boomers of today is that in the past there was a collective consciousness held together by shared noble ideals and virtues to address the wrongs of society that were based on the fears and vulnerabilities of the Greatest Generation's concern for stability and holding on to what had been gained. Today, that collective consciousness has dissipated. Boomers make fewer socially responsible choices in their lives and in their outside associations. The younger generation makes even less.

Yes, there are those individuals—most of whom are boomers—with the courage and outrage to unveil the hoaxes behind the slogans of politicians, financiers, corporate executives, and the media. But let us not forget, the perpetual creators of these hoaxes are boomers, although this awareness has yet to seep into the collective consciousness of the general population. The courageous activist voices of change today, among boomers and young adults alike, remain relatively small. But they represent the next movement, which may take five to ten years to reach a new collective consciousness that will inspire decisive activism. In the meantime, it may very well take a major crisis affecting the majority of the nation's population before anyone will listen.

What I find most sad is that today's young adults, with few exceptions, appear almost oblivious that anything spiritually urgent is happening around them. During my conversation with one of today's more brilliant social historians and critics of contemporary culture, Morris Berman told me that at the time of the Iraq war, approximately 18 percent of young adults could not find Iraq on the map. In his important work, *The Twilight of American Culture,* Morris discusses a little-known study revealing that a notable number of young adults were unable to even locate the United States on a map. Ask most members of the younger generation what the First Amendment and habeas corpus mean or about the effects of the Patriot Act and you will receive a blank stare. And who can be blamed for their ignorance about the world and the purpose of life except the boomers and the society they have built?

I would like readers of this book, whether a boomer, a senior citizen, or a young adult who is just entering society as a productive citizen, to consider one of two fundamental choices that will shape and guide your life.

The first choice is to remain unwilling to change and stay as we are, as servants to the existing social paradigm and the powers that control it. If our attitude is to get through life now and not feel any connection with or responsibility toward the society around us, then we will continue to be myopic and whine and complain about the injustices we witness. We are only able to be beneficial and constructive members of our society, as well as of the global community, if we take ownership of our role and responsibility in preserving the best they have to offer. Therefore it is incumbent upon us to understand how every choice we make affects someone, somewhere, and every day.

If I decide to watch an inane reality program, I am participating in the station's ratings and contributing to the program's ratings and survival. If I acquiesce to a child's desires to have a hamburger or french fries in a McDonald's, then my money is like casting a personal vote saying I favor and support junk food. If I work for a corporation whose consumer products I know are detrimental to the well-being and health of another person, then I am directly responsible for inflicting disease upon them. Therefore, we need to take an eagle's eye view of our entire lives and decide for ourselves whether we are healing our world or making it more ill. If our decision is to do nothing, then we will continue to run the rat race and fall victim to others who do not care for our best spiritual interests and personal growth.

The alternative choice is to commit ourselves to awakening and learning to become aware of our exchange of energies with ourselves and each other. If we become accountable for our thoughts, our words, and our deeds, and then realize the positive or negative effects these have upon our authentic self, we can begin to live virtuous lives. Physical reality—our society, nation, and the planet—is determined by how we act, for better or worse. If want to improve our society, we must become honest with ourselves and then challenge the status quo.

During the 1960s and early 1970s, young boomers tried to walk their talk. They were unafraid of taking the risk of standing out by standing up. They were committed to their ideals and to their vision of a better and more free society. So I believe it is time for boomers to become "hippies" again. I do not mean to don tie-dyed clothes and deny themselves the wonderful inventions modern society has created to bring comfort into our lives. Instead, I mean boomers should reclaim the vitality that has been lost over the past three decades. In this way, boomers can create new communities and visions during their remaining years and share that vitality with their children's generation, which is hungering for something more meaningful than the ceaseless pursuit of possessions, a better paycheck, and pleasures that disappear immediately after they are experienced.

The choice is ours to make. And our choices will determine the legacy we leave for our children. Will it be a legacy that lives and breathes new meaning into society or will it be a legacy best left in the grave?

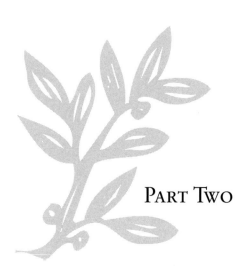

PART TWO

CHAPTER TWO

Embracing Our Bliss

We're going to explore something that I first heard about in Bill Moyers' PBS series, *Joseph Campbell and the Power of Myth*. Campbell talked about bliss. That's not a concept that I grew up with, so I began to wonder, "What is bliss? What does it mean?" What keeps us from our bliss? What manifests bliss?

Bliss is about having the courage to release immature notions that make us toxic to ourselves and others. I began to understand that bliss has more to do with what we must undo or not do than with what we must do. It's about letting go of fear instead of drawing our defense mechanisms out like samurai swords. When we live in fear we tend to bury our head in the sand indefinitely like an ostrich. While taking a brief vacation to regain perspective can be helpful, like fasting from the news every so often, consistent withdrawal will soon leave you unprepared for the adventure of life as it unfolds.

Success in life is not just about making sound choices; it is often about rejecting choices that may defeat you and others. Compare this to your nutrition choices. By eliminating a few foods from your diet, such as meat, wheat, dairy, and sugar, you could feel better almost immediately. First you must find out what you do on automatic pilot that is harmful.

There are two ways of approaching health. One is to take supplements and add a host of activities that you wouldn't normally do, such as lifting weights. Another approach is to simply stop doing things that destroy health. I find that people who stop doing things that are toxic remain just about as healthy as those who do damaging things and then try to compensate by detoxifying and supplementing. So if you don't smoke, don't drink, don't eat sugar, red meat, or processed foods, you're likely to be about as healthy as someone working very hard to compensate for their bad habits. Removing toxic items from your diet and environment soon improves your health, even if you do nothing else. Apply that same concept to bliss by purging your preconceived notions, or conditioning, that narrow the mind and wreak havoc with your emotional states.

Bliss is a natural state, conditioning is not. Your conditioned responses act as a firewall to separate you from bliss. Bliss is like purity. No baby is ever born with a negative attitude, but over time fear, psychoses, neuroses, depression, and anxiety develop that give rise to limitations, biases, and prejudices, which are conditioned responses. Fortunately, anything that is a result of conditioning can be reversed.

I'm going to ask a series of questions so you can discover your own relationship to embracing your bliss. I'll give you some of my own insights, but that's my own particular view. It is no more valid than yours. It's intended to prod you to think deeply. When you find a quiet moment, reflect and ask yourself what each question means.

First, are you willing to release your conditioned beliefs? We believe many things throughout our lives that may not be true. Sources of false information may include our families, teachers, friends, books, the media, and our own misinterpretation of our experiences.

Once you believe something, are you capable of changing your mind if evidence to the contrary becomes available? A renowned professor was visiting a Zen master, who asked, "Tea?" "Yes," said the professor. The Zen master began to pour the tea, and continued pouring. As the hot tea began to run over the rim of the cup, the professor, shocked, cried, "Enough!" There was nothing that could be added to the professor's cup. When our minds are full of dogma, like "professor-mind," there is no room for fresh knowledge. Keep emptying. Is your cup already full, or are you ready for refreshing new insights?

Do you cling to the notion of permanence to resist change? Life is impermanent. That's not what we believe early in life, however. Teenagers don't worry about impermanence because they do not usually have to come face to face with that impermanence unless they lose a pet or a grandparent dies. They're told what's happening, but it doesn't really register. There is sorrow and there is grief, but buoyancy soon returns.

The older we get, the more impermanence haunts us because we envision death encountering us somewhere on our path, though we never know how or when it will come. We know we cannot escape, yet we try to convince ourselves that we can somehow elude the ultimate change.

If we don't want life to be over, then we will feel betrayed because we didn't desire the end. But once you allow yourself to realize that life is impermanent, you will regret that your lifelong loyalty to the illusion of permanence prevented you from accessing your real self, instead becoming society's cutout pattern of you. We want a permanent home and a permanent job and a permanent relationship because we imagine that we can have a permanent life.

Up until this most recent generation, society enforced the notion that everything was meant to be permanent. Your values were the ideals that you accepted from society's model, which taught you to find one relationship, to have a home and live there forever, to work loyally at one job, and to be obedient to the rules of a society that offered rewards for your compliance.

Then one day when you lose your job you realize that things aren't permanent after all. You think, *Wait a second. I gave you all my trust. I gave you everything. Why don't I get to stay in this job forever?* Until the 1970s, most people took a job thinking that was it; in fact, you were considered irresponsible if you changed jobs. If you had more than two jobs in a lifetime, people would wonder what was wrong with you. Now you might have two jobs a year.

Certain types of people embrace change, and others resist. You can't have both permanence and change. We know in our hearts that nothing ever stays the same; we know that life evolves. The deepest pool will stagnate if there is no circulation. We know that our muscles atrophy if there is no movement, that brain cells die if we don't think and challenge ourselves. Yet the last thing most people want, once they're comfortable with what they're doing, is change. We think change equals pain, which is why so many people who know they could do better and know what needs to change won't take those steps.

One of the problems with the permanence paradigm is that after the establishment tells you that you have a permanent this and a permanent that, you wake up one day and realize that you don't. By then you've already given your loyalty to the permanency illusion, and your loyalty has left you somewhat frustrated. Today even pension funds, once regarded as permanent sacred trusts, are not always safe. You've paid allegiance to something that is not legitimate.

You can honor the system, but unfortunately it does not always honor you. We're faithful to the idea of permanence, but life isn't. Life is always going forward.

Expectation is a conditioned response that often breeds disappointment. Have you ever looked in a mirror and felt sadness when you compare the face in the reflection to your photo from ten years ago on the mantle? You think, *What's wrong with this picture? I'm not supposed to age like this.* Your longstanding expectation that you would remain young breeds disappointment and prevents you from appreciating who you are now. Separation from your youthful self brings a nostalgic loneliness, as if your younger self were now betraying you by disappearing. When you live in the moment and you accept the moment as fleeting, then you don't feel betrayed.

Do you become entangled in your emotions and compare yourself mercilessly to others? The next lesson is: change your emotional leitmotif. Ask yourself which of your feelings discourage you. How you live will create either a positive feeling or a negative feeling that plays through your life like a recurring operatic theme. Once you've established that there's a feeling that undermines you, then you have to ask, *How did I end up manifesting this? Why do I get angry? What makes me angry? How often do I get angry? What do I do when I'm angry? Is it something constructive or destructive that I do with my anger?* Or, you might wonder, *Why am I envious? Am I envious because I'm jealous? Do I feel that what I have or what I am or what I think or what I do is second-rate? Am I always comparing myself to others? Why should I do that? Where does that come from? Did my parents compare me to my siblings, cousins, or schoolmates? Did my teachers compare me to other students? Did I compare my grades*

*to Bobby's? Did my coach compare me with my teammates? Or were
the comparisons more subtle, barely traceable, perhaps? Why can't
I just accept that whatever I am and whatever I feel is me?*

The trouble is, we don't question how we become tangled in
these emotional critiques. There is a fine line between *objective comparison,* which is a detached, detailed observation of differences and
similarities with no emotional component, and *judgmental criticism,*
which may be severe, hostile, disapproving, faultfinding, and often
emotional. If you've been primed from childhood to judge things
and people, including yourself, harshly (even if camouflaged by
humor), the only way to stop is to become aware of the condemnation. Take notice.

Bliss disappears when your negative emotions surge. How often do
you feel these emotions? Most importantly, what are the consequences of negative emotions? When you engage in envy, fear, jealousy, worry, and anger, there's always a consequence to yourself first.
You stay attached to everything you create. So if you're worrying
about someone, you're also the victim of that worry. If you're angry
with someone, you're also the victim of your own anger. Everything
you try to send out there clings to you automatically.

You could have all those emotions in one day. None of them are
constructive. How do you get that way? In part because you lack
the ability to see life for what it is, and to see people for who they are.

Zen Buddhism places great emphasis on surrendering the belief
that you are "special" so that you can revel in the most "ordinary"
simple joys of life, which you now barely notice—a breeze, a walk,
an orange, a smile, washing your hands. In Zen, these are just as
special as you are, because they *are* you. These drab peahens of life
suddenly become peacocks displaying a feast of riches before you,
but only when you relate simply to the ordinary objects, people, and

moments of life as they appear—not when you are focused superficially on how special you are, and how inferior (or superior) others are by comparison.

A humane ethical life means respect for others. Albert Schweitzer, MD (1875–1965), the Alsatian physician-theologian-philosopher, was a peace activist who received the Nobel Peace Prize in 1952 for his philosophy of "reverence for life," which he expressed in many ways, but which is especially well reflected in his founding of the Lambaréné Hospital in Gabon, West Central Africa, in 1913. Schweitzer taught that society is "full of folly" that will deceive us about consideration for the lives and happiness of others. Respect for life, resulting from contemplation of one's own will to live, leads us to live to serve other people and every living being. Dr. Schweitzer found many ways, big and small, to put his theory into practice in his daily life. For example, Schweitzer was left-handed, but he would write with his right hand rather than awaken the cat who loved to sleep on his left arm.

Jack Paar, the 1950s talk-show host, used to tell of a visit he took to Dr. Schweitzer's hospital in Africa. One day as they walked down the road, the doctor abruptly ceased conversing and stopped in his tracks. A caterpillar was slowly crossing the road, endangering herself. Dr. Schweitzer knelt down and gently lifted the caterpillar, depositing her safely at her destination. He then continued the conversation as if nothing had happened. He did this all the time, apparently, thinking it a routine kindness. No celebrity was going to distract Dr. Schweitzer from his characteristic generosity.

Slow down and reconnect with relationships. We have become a nation destitute of strong relationships. There is too much stimulation and too much busyness; so little time, so many malls. We need to slow down and learn from the life we live. We need to learn to stop overcluttering our lives and seeking perfection, and to become more nurturing in our relationships.

We have the ability to look at our history, culture, and institutions to see what mistakes we have made as a society, and as individuals within society. The same errors that cause us to fail as a nation doom us as families and as individuals. The moment we abandon eternal truths, either individually or collectively, we fail. So let us discover what once worked; old lessons can be brought back as new. Do not steal. Do not lie. Do not cheat. These commandments are just as life-giving as they were when they were received. We are meant to apply these in all of our relationships; they tell us how to interact with one another peaceably.

Although my parents were not the best models for health, I was fortunate to have been deeply influenced by a dynamic catalyst, my great aunt, who ran a farm and knew everything about it, in silent dialogue with her partner, the earth. You've heard of a "horse whisperer." Well, my aunt had that kind of a subtle, powerful relationship with the land. They were close. Their fellowship was not mystical exactly because it was so practical, but you wondered how she knew so much about it all, with that way she had of just looking up at the sky and squinting sometimes, listening for the wind, or for the rain before it came. We usually lose those intuitive instincts before we hit our teens. If you keep them alive, they can lead you to a healthy, perceptive life.

Once you eat "real food" like my great aunt's, once you've bitten into a fresh, ripe flavorful tomato, then tasteless genetically modified crops with their mushy waterlogged tomatoes are a sacrilege. Texture and taste are gone; it's unnatural. That's where I learned to regard a healthy lifestyle as essential. I was fortunate that there was a human catalyst, a great earth teacher, in my family to guide me to a wholesome appreciation for the land, the water, and the air. The Cherokee roots in my family led me to the natural law of "always give back." If you use wood to build a fire, use the gift of fire, then give the wood, as ashes, back to the earth by burying them in a self-sustaining pattern of gratefulness.

Working on the farm was hard work, but it was worth it. I am still devoted to the healthy lifestyle I learned there. I use the same organic farming principles on my ranch today, where I grow a full range of varieties of vegetables and fruits, which sustain my family, guests, and staff. Everything I grow is certified organic produce, and I also sell it at a farmers market, so to a small degree it helps sustain healthy minds in the community.

Free yourself from the traps of materialism. Unclutter your life. Many impulsive shoppers buy things they seldom use. This is, in fact, considered to be a sign that you may be either a shopaholic or a hoarder.

On the contrary, as I mentioned at the start, eliminating things is most often what leads us back to bliss, which is our original state before we load up on nonessentials that obscure our mental clarity, as clouds hide the sun. Brilliance and economy are often linked because nature, in its wisdom, wastes nothing.

A reporter who once interviewed Albert Einstein noticed he had a shaving cut on his face. "Professor Einstein," the reporter said, "what kind of shaving soap do you use?" "*Shaving* soap?" Einstein asked. "Yes," the reporter continued, "you have a special soap that you use when you shave, don't you?" Einstein thought for a moment and asked incredulously, "*Two* soaps?" The thought of using anything extra was absurd to a scientist used to calculating energy expenditure in a universe that conserves everything. Einstein, by the way, rode the subway (you may recall his interest in trains) with his brown-bag lunch. He did not even bother to buy what he *could* afford.

Consider whether you are embracing bliss or a tiger when you make your next credit card purchase, which means you are going into debt to obtain property, food, or remedies that you may not even need.

Prepare for opportunity. If you were presented with a unique opportunity, would you be prepared to engage it? How many times in life has opportunity arrived, but you weren't prepared so you had to pass? The one thing you can start doing now is to prepare yourself for anything. Then you're going to create opportunity. The more prepared you are and the more open you are, the more chances will come your way. If you do not participate because of fear that you're not ready or aren't good enough and will fail, you will be stuck sitting on the sidelines of life. You become the passive spectator watching everybody else in action, saying, "That looks like so much fun. Why am I not doing that?"

So prepare yourself emotionally, spiritually, physically, intellectually, and creatively. Take every part of your life that needs sharpening and start honing. Focus and unclutter so that when the opportunity appears, you're ready to go.

You may never find bliss if you follow someone else's goals, and misery may await you. When you select a goal, ask yourself, *Is this my goal, or is it someone else's?* Your bliss depends on your answer. As often as not, the goals you pursue are someone else's hand-me-downs that they passed on to you. They may, in turn, have received their goals from someone else. Your father's goal for you to become a hero by following him and his forebears into a lifetime career in the military may have originally belonged to your great-grandfather. You've got to relinquish everyone else's goals for you, unless their suggested goal coincides with your own. That happens sometimes, but not always.

Tackle one goal at a time. In order to achieve your goal you must have a long-term strategy. Pace yourself with small, slow steps. Be very patient. Do not allow yourself to be distracted by other agendas. People today are frequently distracted. We even go out of our way to be distracted because if something is distracting us then we can always use the excuse that we don't have the time to work on ourselves. We're too busy and have too many things to do. *Don't blame me if I never get anything done.* We're not going to blame you. We're also going to say, *Don't make any more excuses.*

Aim at one single thing, and that's it. Nothing else. Make it the thing that you really want, that will mean something when you achieve it. Take that one meaningful thing and add it to your life and do not allow any other distraction. It is the distraction of multiple tasks and responsibilities that undermines you. It can be self-defeating. We know that if we take on more than what we can do, we're going to limit ourselves. Then we can quit by saying that there is too much to do.

Love has the power to bring you bliss by positively transforming your reactions to the challenges in your life. The Roman poet Virgil said that love conquers all. When you use love to meet a challenge or overcome an obstacle, you embrace bliss. What do we normally use to overcome obstacles? Fear, anger, uncertainty, envy, or jealousy. Think of how many times you've been motivated by jealousy. What if, instead, you simply had love? Do you know what love can do to a problem? It transforms your reaction to it. Love guides you to reframe events and give the benefit of the doubt to yourself and others.

Love is not a fool's paradise, though; it's more practical than that. It's hard to fight someone when you have love. It's easy when you have anger. That's the power of love. Love has to come from you. You have to keep accessing it and allowing it.

Activism is generosity, our universal calling. Honor your dharma as a permanent goal. The Sanskrit word for duty is *dharma,* which also means teaching and truth. Isn't it our duty as human beings to teach the love that we have for life, and the interest we have in all things, and how connected we are even though we have been conditioned to believe that we're so uniquely different? What distinguishes us as human beings is our ability to have an affinity for another person, no matter what their age, race, or religion may be. If you extend that humane quality to others, then you are honoring the duty of your life. You are honoring your dharma. You're sharing the truth that we are all more alike and more equal than we would like to believe.

Each moment is all you have. When moments are all we have, how do we choose what to do with each moment? We can focus on what's important or we can distract ourselves with the unimportant. How much of your time is spent on unimportant moments? Most of the time, if we really examine our lives, we're doing the nonessential. Live in the moment.

In all you do, your intention matters. When offering anything that we have, it's our intention that is important, not the size or significance of the offering. People will often not contribute what they can because they think they don't have anything that is significant enough. *Other* *people can give more. They're wiser or richer. What do I have? I'm just a nobody.* Not true. Yes, there are people who always give a big gift. Everybody then announces they've done it, and we all applaud. Do not compare yourself to them.

Sometimes we have no idea how much a timely gift can mean to someone. Graciela worked for an architecture firm. She was a divorced mom with three young children to support. Her boss, Mr. H., president of the company, was a difficult man to work for. Graciela was his secretary, and she worked very hard. She was always putting in extra hours. Graciela's generosity and cheerfulness was appreciated by everyone in the office, except her boss. For a woman who desperately needed her job, his indifference was of concern to Gracie.

As the year was coming to a close, Gracie wondered if she would be fired or get a raise, or a bonus. She'd been there two years, and Mr. H. had never praised her, not once. Suddenly, it was Christmas Eve. It was almost five o'clock, and it was snowing.

Mr. H. left his office with his coat and hat on, nodded to Gracie, brusquely said, "Merry Christmas," and quickly left. It took a moment, but Gracie realized that Mr. H. did not intend to give her any personal gift. Her eyes filled with tears as the fact that there would be no token of his appreciation began to sink in. "What did you get from Ebenezer?" Lana asked. "Nothing," Gracie answered. "What?" Lana asked incredulously.

Just then the bookkeeper, Jerry, began to distribute the checks that would reveal a raise or bonus. Jerry said, "Merry Christmas, Gracie," as he handed her the envelope. *What if I cry?* she thought. Gracie went into Mr. H.'s office to open the envelope. *I'll be safer in here where it's more private.* Gracie opened her envelope. There was no pink slip. Her check was for the usual amount. There was no bonus check enclosed, and no raise listed. Gracie didn't cry. She was becoming angry. She decided to quit. She would tell Jerry, collect all her things, and go.

Just then, Mr. Wan, an architect who had recently started working at the firm, knocked on the open door to Mr. H.'s office. "May I come in?" he asked. "Oh, sure," Gracie answered quietly. "This is for you, Gracie," he said, "Merry Christmas," presenting her with a small package wrapped in bright red paper, and tied with a gold ribbon. Gracie smiled. "Why, thank you, Mr. Wan." "Ted. My name's Ti-Hua, but my friends call me Ted." "Thank you, Ted."

Gracie pulled opened the golden ribbon and the shiny red paper. Inside was a black satin pouch with gorgeous bright flowers embroidered on it. "It's from China," Ted said, enthusiastically. Gracie reached into the satin pouch to find a small black-and-gold flacon of perfume. On the vial was one word painted in gold script, *Zen*. She almost expected a genie to emerge from the bottle. A beautiful scent. "It's just Shiseido," he added. "Will you have a Christmas Eve toast with me at the Top of the Rock?" Gracie was overwhelmed. She nodded yes. "Thank you, Ted, thank you. What a beautiful gift." Ted smiled.

Gracie went to get her coat and noticed that Jerry had already gone home, so there was no way she could quit, even if she'd wanted to. Better to think it over, anyway. Her kids were with Grandma, so she had time for the drink. It occurred to Gracie that if she hadn't been hit so hard and been made so vulnerable by her boss, she might not have been as receptive to Ted's invitation. She'd been pretty wary since her divorce. Something good was happening here.

"Ready?" Ted asked, as he appeared in his coat and dashing fedora. *Oh, he's so handsome,* Gracie noticed. Ted's gift was a modest one. But it was well-timed, and romantic. Its effect was immeasurable. It changed their lives forever, for the better.

The poor can be as generous as the rich, and as blissful, or more so. On a cold, rainy Sunday evening in March when Frank arrived at the church, the last of the free dinners for the homeless and destitute had already been served. He'd just missed a great hot meal of lasagna with Italian green beans, fresh salad, garlic bread, and home-baked red velvet cake with freshly brewed hot tea. Frank had never been to St. Malachy's before. He was new on the needy circuit. He'd never had a free meal in his life, but he sure needed one now. Down on his luck for the first time, it wasn't easy for him to show up for this.

He had intended to arrive early, but he'd stopped to chat with a friend who was in trouble, so he was late, and he was hungry. "Sorry, sir," said Carmen, the hostess at the door. "Nothing left." "Nothing?" asked Frank, alarmed. Just then, Anthony, all the way in the back of the dining room, realized Frank's plight and held up a cling-wrapped sandwich from St. Francis' church and yelled, "Peanut butter and jelly okay?" Frank's face lit up as he rushed toward the sandwich. "Thanks," he said. "Okay," said Anthony. Then Eddie piped up with a Hostess apple pie and a banana. "Over here, pal," said Eddie. Frank thanked Eddie. "I gotta sugar-free butterscotch pudding and an apple," Buddy called out. "Great," said Frank, "Thanks."

Soon Frank had a whole meal, plus unlimited tea and juice. It was a meal he'd never forget because it was truly communal, a family-style rescue, without any obligation. Frank could hardly believe it. He felt welcome.

Next time he would bring something to share, although it was not required. No one would keep score. Until he could get back on his feet, Frank, a total stranger, would not go hungry at St. Malachy's, or anywhere that big hearts gather gratefully at humanity's generous table.

Moments are not meant for recapture, but are to be replaced. Like our own cells, moments must be allowed to die to make way for fresh new life. At some point in life when you're quiet, you realize that moments are not meant to be recaptured, but rather to be replaced. Prepare in the present to be open and vulnerable for the next moment.

We enjoy something that touches us and something that resonates with our essential self; it manifests bliss. We say, *this is so good.* It is. And, let it go. It stays with you in the energy you shared and the memory of that energy. That will be with you for eternity, but if you stay focused on trying to recapture it, you close yourself off to another unique and precious moment. You must be prepared for the next moment, and to be prepared for it, you must surrender the moment you're in so you're not living in the past. You're present. Being present allows you to have another blissful moment or another painful moment, but at least you are in the moment. That too will pass. Let it go. Moments must be permitted to die in order to yield to fresh new moments. In time, if you do this, your life will be filled with renewable joy.

The adventure of changing the world begins first with surrendering your fear so you can be yourself. When you feel sad, angry, or helpless, how often do you blame the world? The world isn't at fault. The problem is that you're not allowing your authentic self to be present to make choices that can help our world. Remember, we can all make a difference, but we can't make a difference out there until we make a difference inside. The conditioning that separates you from yourself and from your bliss is also what alienates us from each other. The journey of changing the world starts first with surrendering your fear so you can be who you are. Every human being has bliss inside waiting to be recognized and embraced.

Learn to be patient and comfortable with uncertainty because freedom from fear brings bliss. It has been said that patience is the master virtue because if you have acquired the habit of being patient, all other virtues will follow more readily. If we think of patience as the palm, other virtues such as kindness, courage, and humility are the fingers that will radiate naturally from that palm of patience.

Charles and Helen were a young married couple from New York City who went to live and teach on an Native American reservation in the Southwest. They had a vegetable patch in which they had planted the trinity of native crops: corn, beans, and squash.

Early every morning, nervous Charles would rush outside to check and see if the beans had sprouted. He was secretly afraid that the Native Americans, great stewards of the earth, would laugh at their new teacher if he was a farming failure. Helen, watching from their hut window, noticed that Charles would quickly brush away the soil to check on the roots. She finally said to him, "Don't you have any patience? You're going to kill those beans if you don't give them a chance to grow." Helen was astounded that she was having to tell an Ivy League graduate not to dig up seeds if he wanted them to grow.

Charles was not at ease with uncertainty, but he promised Helen he'd leave the beans alone for a week. He threw himself into teaching, began to enjoy his classes, and started to relax and feel welcome. Helen was now tending the garden, so he didn't go to peek at any roots.

A week later, the beanstalks were shooting up out of the ground. Charles never engaged in the self-defeating behavior of clawing at seeds again. His trust and patience were growing along with those roots. A few months later, Helen announced that they were going to have a baby. When Helen's doctor asked them if they would like to know the sex of their baby before birth, Charles looked at Helen, smiled, and said calmly, "No, doctor, that won't be necessary." Charles had realized that, as a result of his social conditioning, he'd begun to hope for a boy to impress the tribe because he mistakenly thought they'd think him more macho with a son. Charles, now the brave captain of his own awareness, had become more friendly with uncertainty, and he was embracing bliss.

Once you know bliss, you'll never want to go back to the pain and limitation of a life of sublimation, complacency, and impatience. Just to belong, or to be recognized by others as okay, is no longer enough; it's too shallow. Only when you step beyond your conditioning and let yourself pass through the fear, loneliness, and uncertainty of what will take conditioning's place can bliss embrace you.

What is bliss? Supreme joy, unencumbered. **What prevents us from embracing bliss?** Turmoil. Our conditioned responses, including fear, that make us biased and hypercritical. Younger children know bliss all the time, without seeking it, because their conditioning is still minimal. As adults, it may be difficult for us to experience bliss because we are polluted with prejudices, preconceived notions, guilt, and mistrust, all of which obscure joy. So clear a path for profound appreciation that transcends understanding. Don't limit yourself; contribute. Some of us find bliss helping out in a soup kitchen. Discover what brings you that peace and contentment.

When you know bliss, then everything is possible because you're complete. You're conquering or at least taming the dragon of conditioning that was obstructing your view by becoming aware of your conditioned responses. Keep noticing them; remain vigilant because conditioned responses are like weeds that can grow back. You'll never return to the prison of an overgrown jungle of ignorance if you keep pruning.

How do I embrace bliss? Let bliss embrace you. It finds you when you're not looking for it, if you allow yourself to be open, loving, and vulnerable, instead of closed, selfish, and judgmental.

Bliss cannot be forced; you can only prepare yourself, in openness, to receive it. Like love, it is a gift that comes to those who are ready to welcome it.

CHAPTER THREE

How to Manifest a Beautiful Life

All of us want a beautiful life. We want lovely objects around us and wonderful thoughts, and we want to be in beautiful places. In this chapter we're going to explore what we can do to actualize these desires.

When I say *beauty,* I mean beauty on a spiritual level, on an emotional level, and even on a physical level. How often has your image in the mirror upset you because you didn't like what you saw? How did you get that way? How did you begin to fall apart physically? We think: *Okay, I'm older. Shouldn't I look older?* Up to a point, yes. But if we believe we should, our belief will create our reality. Much of what you believe you are will manifest. Sometimes it happens subtly; you're not even aware of what you're thinking.

One of our problems is that we don't know where to begin our journey. In reality, everyone can start, at any time and any place. Whether you're rich or poor, educated or not, you can still start your journey to create a beautiful life. Let's see what steps you can take to get there.

1. Stay Completely Present

The very first step in any journey is to stay absolutely and completely present. What if you could visualize your body a year from now just by staying present and looking at yourself? Ask yourself: *How could I have that body a year from now?* By being present and resting in your quiet, feeling mind, you can detach from everything, seeing everyone and everything for what they are. Your awareness allows you to understand what you're doing or what you would do, and the consequences. Then you can say: *All right. Now that I see this I can make a more informed and reasonable choice.*

No one likes to look back and think: *Did I make all those stupid things happen?* Yes. Could they have been different? Yes. Why weren't they different? Because you were stuffing too much into every moment to pay attention to what the moment could have really meant. We tend to think that as long as we're doing our work well, being responsible and on time, that those things are a good use of our time. But are they really? What if you used your time to honor your life?

2. To Honor Your Life You Have to Be Aware That You Have a Life

We know we have responsibilities. We know we have relationships. We know we have jobs. But do we know we have a life? Some people don't know that because they don't slow down long enough, they don't go to that neutral place that will allow them to realize the consequences of not having a life. What they feel and what they're emoting are the consequences of the choices they've made, as if someone is sticking them with a pin every other minute. We tend to adjust to this state of affairs, and before we know it, our whole life involves limiting the pain, the hassles, and the stresses of each day instead of paying attention to the uniqueness of each day. You *can* make different choices. You don't have to be stuck, and you don't have to have the pain. You don't have to be caught up in your own busyness.

You can slow yourself down. You can ask yourself: *Why am I doing this? Why am I saying that? Why am I eating that? Why am I having the same phone conversation for the hundredth time? Why am I spilling out my guts when it will change nothing?* You can confess your life and your problems one thousand times over to everybody who wants to listen, and they'll cry with you; you can put yourself on the journey of finding someone who will suffer with you and who will bear witness to your suffering; but what really changes? Little to nothing. How many people want to share pleasure compared to those who want to share suffering? Isn't it amazing? There are no limits to what you can tell a person when it comes to your suffering, but what you can say about your pleasure is so very circumscribed. We've got it all wrong. Make a point to share your positive energy and pleasure, and see what happens.

3. *Our Illusions of Identity*

If we work at a certain job and earn a certain amount of money, we can buy a certain type of clothes, usually expensive. But do your clothes define you as a better person? No, that's an illusion. We can live in a fancy apartment, we can eat in fancy restaurants, not necessarily better, but perceived as better because they're more expensive and more unique. We might even get wealthy enough to be invited to exclusive places by people considered to be elite, but the idea that they're better is an illusion too.

I counsel all types of people. I counsel some of the wealthiest and most famous people and also some of the poorest people in New York, and I want to tell you something I have noticed. People have a very specific idea of their value. More often than not their value is based on what they possess, on their reputation, or on what they've achieved. Everywhere you look we're trying to separate people by such illusions, and eventually we get a collective mindset by which people believe in a common illusion together.

We believe the rich are more valuable than the poor. We believe the educated are more valuable than the uneducated. We believe the person who goes to church is more valuable than the person who doesn't. We think a married person is more valuable than a single person. We think the person who is older is more valuable than the younger person irrespective of who they are (unless they're *too* old, and then they're not valuable at all).

It takes courage to step aside and say no to these illusions. Only you can decide what's real and what's illusory.

4. *All of Our Beliefs Hold Conditioning*

We are conditioned to accept the content of our beliefs. Let's say you're on a subway and someone smiles at you. The content of the conditioning around that smile is: *Don't look at a stranger, especially on a subway. You're going to put yourself at risk. Look down. Look away.* But if you discover something on your own instead of relying on your preconceived notions, then you might well change your mind. What if someone smiled at you and you smiled back? To get rid of your conditioning you have to realize that the conditioning is there because it holds a lot of content that is constantly being reloaded with old messages over and over again. Every time you hear the same message, it reinforces what you've already been told. We will stay prisoners to the messages unless we can get to neutral, to that quiet place where we can examine the messages and ask ourselves which ones are biased, which ones are unfair, and which ones lack honesty and objectivity. You've got to reach that place in your life where you can look at something and say, *No, I don't believe it any more.* When you disconnect right then and there from those messages, you will begin to discover your freedom.

5. Discover the Flow of Your Life

How many times have we pulled our energy back when we might have allowed ourselves to flow forward? You can block your own energy or you can let the energy flow. Everything in life is about constricting or flowing. Let me give you an example. We look at our bank balance and see that we've overspent. The first thing we do is constrict. We start feeling insecure because there's a shortage. We can't buy what we want. We lack abundance, which makes us apprehensive and makes us overreact. We fight with anyone else who may have participated in our overspending: *Why did we buy that? We can't afford it!*

Or people say: *I don't have a life any more. All I'm doing is working to pay my bills. I'm living in New York City. I can't enjoy the city because I have to work so hard. By the time I get home at night I'm tired. So I hang out with other people who also live in New York City who are frustrated by what they can't afford and we kvetch and complain together.* Who put you here? Why don't you look for another place to live? Because instead of opening up, you close down.

The moment any stimulus from our environment says there is a shortage—of money or love or respect—we constrict. We get tight in the stomach. You know what I'm talking about—something isn't right, and you feel it in your gut. You get headaches and you get strains in your back and neck. We constrict because we can't control people or the outcome of events. We get overwhelmed by our circumstances. On top of the circumstances, there are all those voices in our heads telling us how we should react and how we should respond. Visualize that you're in a lifeboat. You're in a rough patch of water. You have a paddle, but you can't control the boat because the current is too strong. You force yourself onward because you see an island, and you think that's what you need. But the closer you get to the island, the more apparent it becomes that it's not a lush, beautiful, bountiful paradise. It is a barren little outpost. But you're thinking: *It's something, it's better than nothing.* So you put all your energy into getting there. While the current is still pulling you away, you jump out of the boat and start swimming. Now your single purpose is to get to safety, and you do. You get up on the beach. You look around and think, *I'm glad I'm out of the water. I'm glad I'm out of the current.* But where are you? You look around and see a barren island.

How many times have you chosen a barren relationship, or job, or living environment, or friendship because it was better to choose something in the moment from fear and insecurity? At least you didn't have to concern yourself with the current of life. But now the current of life continues to flow. It's going right by you. Every day the current is flowing, and you're a spectator. You're not in it. What would have happened if you had gone with the current? Where would the current have taken you? How many times have we gone against the current of our own being? You know you should do A, but you're conditioned to do B. You know you should be open to the moment, but you're restricted and uptight. You go against your own internal chi, your own natural self. You're fighting it because the conditioned self is conditioned from a place of fear. And fear will always win if we give in to it. Then you're living on a barren little island.

For a moment in time, you're protected and secure. But whenever you need to feel secure, it means you're moving from insecurity, and when you do that, you'll never fill the void. You'll always feel empty and remain stuck. But what happens if you let yourself flow instead? Where will that current take you? What if it takes you to a place of beauty and harmony and serenity? What if it takes you to where all your own rhythms are flowing with the rhythm of life?

Then you're going to connect with like-minded people, because similar energies always connect. But we're afraid of who we are, and we're afraid of what would happen if we just flow. Take a look at your life and ask yourself how many times you have ended up on a barren little island.

When I go down to Florida I see gated communities everywhere. They are barren islands with golf, tennis, pools, and palm trees. They are closed off from the rest of the world. The inhabitants say: *We don't want anything outside these gates. Stay out, world, and we'll stay in.* You don't have to live in a gated community to be isolated. You can be anywhere and isolate yourself. And when you do there's nothing there for you except your fear. That's the only coat you can put on each day: fear. That's what happens when we make the wrong choice.

That's also what happens when we don't listen to the voice of the internal self, the real self. We listen to the conditioned voices: *You can't do that. You're not rich enough. You're not wise enough. You're too old.* So you think: *I guess that's right. I don't see anybody else doing it, and there are a lot of people like me. Fat. Old. Sad. Depressed. We'll all watch Oprah together.*

What happens if you decide to strike out on your own? The others will ask, Where are you going? *I'm going on with my life.* Hold on a second. What about us? *I'm leaving this island.* You can't leave this island. *Sure I can.* No, you can't. You worked so hard to justify getting here and being here. You were cynical and negative. You made almost all your decisions from fear. We did too. We're your friends. *I don't need friends like you.* You don't know what's out there. *You're right. I don't. But I do know what's here. And I'd rather take the unknown and be in the flow of my life than the known and have no life.* Never make the mistake of confusing your work and your lifestyle with a life.

When you're in the flow of your life you can discover what happens when you expand love and when you give love. What happens when you don't limit the love you give? What happens when you don't fear giving love? Everyone and everything will feel that love. It's wonderful to feel the expansion of love. It keeps on vibrating, and when you connect with something as authentic as unconditional love, you know it. Every human being understands what love is because we were all born as pure love. No baby has ever been born evil or angry or jealous or full of rage. Not one.

When we go against our true selves because of conditioning, we can't trust authentic love. We don't trust the truth and reality of what we could and should be and were meant to be. Instead, we trust the superficial, controlled, manipulated self. We can change that. You have to get off the island of your life to do it. You can't have that love and be on that island. You can't quiet your mind and be on that island. You can't be in the most barren place in your life, no matter how secure it is, and expect a life of any meaning or joy.

6. Distractions Dissipate Energy

How much of your day is spent in distraction? When we put our energy out *there,* it distracts us from what's in *here.* We're always looking out and almost never looking in. We'll overeat, or take tranquilizers, or keep ourselves constantly busy to fill the emptiness of our lives. We can't stay with it. So at the end of the day we don't feel anything except our busyness, and then our minds and all those conditioned voices will say: *You're keeping busy. You've got a to-do list. See, every day you get through ten to fifteen items. You're doing the right thing.*

But what happens if you drop all these balls to just be present for a moment? Look carefully at your life, because only you can decide what your distractions are. Write them all down. Then add up how much time you give to each one. How do these distractions affect you emotionally, intellectually, creatively, physically, and spiritually? Do they enhance you or do they deplete you, and to what degree? How does the depletion manifest? You have the right to stop distracting yourself and regain your energy. When you're focused on the authentic, you're energized. When you're focused on distractions, you're drained.

7. We Can Stop Clinging to Everything and Everybody

All this clinging. All this need for possession. All this need to have someone and something that is yours and unique: it's an illusion. In this world the only thing that you have that's unique to you is yourself. Everything else is just a passage. So enjoy the passages; enjoy the people, enjoy the events. But be present for your life in the moment you're in so you can start making the right choices. Choose the lessons you want to learn.

You have to believe enough in yourself to stop clinging to fear and insecurity, to that sense of *I'm going to be without, I won't have enough,* as if there's a shortage. These are all self-imposed shortages. There is no shortage of love. There is no shortage of experiences. There is no shortage of wonderful people. There is no shortage of beautiful places. There is no shortage of creativity. But you have to believe in yourself. If you want your mind to be creative, you have to challenge your mind. If you want your body to be healthy, you have to feed your body. If you want your soul to be expressive, you have to give unconditional love to the world. You can't do it with fear because fear is going to push you back in the closet, slam the door, and tell you to wait five more years.

Why should we wait one moment? We're alive this second, and we should honor this second. I don't want to wait until all the pieces are together, until all the questions are answered and all my fears have abated, until all my uncertainties have been calmed and all my illusions dispelled. None of us need that in order to declare ourselves open for life.

8. Release Your Energy into Positive Change

I meet people all the time who say *I'm too old to change. I'm too tired to change.* In every human being, there is a dynamic life force. If you keep it controlled and repressed, it won't express itself. Open yourself up to express the dynamic energy that's uniquely your own. It has your signature written all over it. When you connect with that exuberance and start to open up, you're like a beautiful unfolding flower. Suddenly you think: *Wow! This is a wonderful way to feel. I feel free. I'm not making my decisions from fear or limitation or illusion or conditioned self. I'm in the moment. I want to be part of the flow of my life. I'm present for the flow of my life. I don't have to wait until everything is right, until I have enough money or enough support. I'm my own support. Money is not what supports me. Faith in myself supports me. Trusting in that eternal spirit is what I need.*

It's not about your job or your friends or your possessions. It's about starting your journey with one step, but that step shouldn't be a step *forward*. It should be a step *away* from distraction, from busyness, from judging, and from the emotions you use to protect yourself. Go to that empty space where your mind and spirit are present to bear witness. When you bear witness nonjudgmentally, you see everything for what it is, and that's how you make clear choices. Surrender this, engage that. Choose this, reject that: as long as you stay in that neutral and quiet space, everything will flow naturally and effortlessly. Having and manifesting a beautiful life starts with appreciating how much beauty already exists in your life—all you have to do is surrender to it and open up.

CHAPTER FOUR

Living an Illuminated Life

Most of us have heard the term "illumination" in self-help and spiritual literature. Illumination occurs when we are open to all the potential we inherently possess. When the self is open to its full potential, the world is presented before us with great clarity. Each and every one of us has experienced flashes of illumination, truly remarkable moments in our lives, but most of us believe we can only hope to bump into those moments, as if they are out there waiting for us. In this chapter I will offer you the fundamentals for increasing such moments so that each day can be a remarkable experience.

At a ranch I once owned north of Dallas, where the crisp atmosphere was undisturbed by city lights or pollution, the sky often held magnificent cloud formations and exquisite sunsets, giving the sensation of immensity and expansion. When you are alone with that vast sky overhead, free of stress and worry, free from conversations and distractions, there is a feeling of oneness with your environment around you, just you connecting with the consciousness of the moment you are in. That is an example of a remarkable moment of illumination. Just as attempting to describe the sky's immensity, cloud patterns, and far-reaching sunsets to someone else can't convey your experience, so it is with all our moments of illumination. We have to show up for the experiences ourselves.

When do we have a remarkable moment? It might happen when we are with someone we are overwhelmingly enamored by. There is an exchange that takes place when we share energy with a person we love. Although the exchange is invisible, we know it is real because that energy makes us vibrate. We feel it move throughout our body. There may even be moments when that experience returns to us when we are alone and thinking of our loved one. These are remarkable moments connecting us to authentic reality.

A fundamental law of the universe is that it never forgets our experiences. The level at which every cell and molecule in our body vibrates depends upon both the nature of the moment we are in and the memory of every other moment we have ever experienced. Every cell and molecule in our bodies is waiting for a sign from our environment, for some word or some gesture, to trigger a moment that brings us to a deeper realization. If a present experience triggers a positive experience from our past, then the energy we receive back is pleasurable.

For example, in recent years PBS television has been bringing back old doo-wop musicians. Why would doo-wop music be popular in the twenty-first century? The programs are popular for those viewers who can remember a special moment in their past when doo-wop music brought them pleasurable experiences. There was a time when doo-wop meant something to them; it might have been a moment of romantic tenderness with a boyfriend or girlfriend while listening to the music on a car radio, or it might be reliving a moment of youthful freedom on the dance floor, feeling life as full of unlimited possibilities. As memories return, the mind relives past events and the feelings associated with those memories.

Where were those memories residing all this time? At the conscious level they are not always present, but in fact they are always present. Every single moment of our lives, everything we have ever done is stored—nothing is ever forgotten and nothing is ever lost. What really matters is the way in which we connect with those memories. We want to connect with the joyful memories; but we also connect with memories we prefer to forget because they were upsetting or traumatic. Experiences that caused us fear, insecurity, anger, or a sense of being violated or unappreciated are also present. Not only are unpleasant memories stored in our cells, they also unconsciously shape much of our daily behavior, so we need to learn how to create these moments that emphasize and build upon our positive experiences. The cumulative effect of remarkable moments opens us up into a state of illumination.

Take a moment to reflect on people you know who have lived an illuminated life. What distinguishes them from us? They are not inherently different from the rest of us, but they appear to be living at a different level of consciousness. They exude qualities of lightness, ease, and being at peace with themselves. They seem to flow through life, and they project an acute awareness of the moment they are in. We can feel positive energy radiating from their presence, even in their writings.

I frequently adopt orphaned baby animals on one of my farms. Because these babies have been abandoned or rejected in one manner or another, it takes a lot of attention and patience before they warm up to you. Suddenly a day arrives when one of them crawls into your lap, kisses you, and expresses contentment in its own unique way. These little creatures connect fearlessly through love. They are not afraid of being dropped or injured because they instinctively know that you will provide them with comfort and joy. The same is true of human infants who have no fear of being dropped by the mother; you can toss them into the air gently and they only laugh and giggle. But if you drop them several times or yell frequently they become afraid. If a toddler does something you disapprove of and you scold and smack him or her, the child will cower or go hide. Eventually the child will fear you. Those traumatic experiences become embedded in the child's cells as memories and it will take considerable effort to overcome the fears that were conditioned by those destructive experiences.

Adults who have been abused, neglected, or denied in their past may hold the energy of those memories tightly, which can constrict their muscles around it. Even their mental constructs—beliefs and judgments about the world—can constrict. If these people lack sufficient remarkable moments in their lives, they may not see the world as a wonderful, positive place with enormous potential for experiencing creative and pleasurable energies but as something threatening and wrathful.

I am sure you have been in the presence of people who seem numb to life. They don't feel anything because they cling to all of their discomfort toward the world. In contrast, we also know people who seem like endless running rivers of love, who are unafraid of opening themselves to life's bounties and becoming vulnerable in order to accept what the universe has to offer. I have found it very interesting to observe that it is only when people make themselves vulnerable that they are able to grow. There is no growth and no authentic feeling toward life when vulnerability is missing. If we live solely with our past pains, allowing tormenting wounds to register in us physically and emotionally, then no matter what we attempt to do, we will not proceed with an openness that enhances growth and illumination. Vulnerability is a crucial initial step toward illumination.

So if we wish to become illuminated—being present to the moment, open, dynamic, loving, and caring—we need to be vulnerable.

In order to prepare ourselves for illumination, we also have to learn to stop constantly trying to escape the emptiness we feel nagging at our lives. The emptiness isn't real, of course, but we don't even allow ourselves the chance to slow down enough discover its illusory nature and the truth of our vibrant connection to the world.

One of the most common ways to avoid facing an empty sensation is to occupy ourselves with something or immerse ourselves in our habitual routines. Everything we do to remain busy, including all of our addictions and dysfunctional behaviors, is based upon anxiety and fear of that emptiness, which we would rather avoid or fill than confront. How we busy ourselves depends upon our earlier conditioning, our intellect, and our unique disposition. For example, some people are afraid of exposing their true motives to others so they present façades to cover up their intentions. They might try to fill their emptiness with beauty, surrounding themselves with beautiful possessions or obsessing about their appearance, but there is a fundamental flaw to such strategies.

Imagine for a moment you are a beautiful person by accepted social standards, but then a day arrives when you realize that your beauty is impermanent. A beauty that only conforms to society's norms is going to end eventually. How are you going to feel when you are no longer accepted for being beautiful? As long as you are desired, beauty is your opium; it puts you into an altered state. Yet deep inside you there is another voice saying, "But only for today." What happens if you have no other value but your beauty to bank on, and then the currency of your glamour runs out? Suddenly you will find yourself starting to maneuver and manipulate in order to connect with someone who is successful and won't care about your beauty's demise. You will then have security to replace the emptiness that you filled earlier with your attachment to being beautiful. This is a scenario I have seen people enact numerous times.

I have also observed how so many men and women today avoid associating with those who are authentically aligned with illuminative qualities, who could offer them a vital connection to something essential. Instead they seek people who will provide or support their needs for security. Security can mean something different for each person. One of the most common manifestations of security is our desire to put down roots with a family and children and own a home. Such pursuits are perfectly fine unless you are tied to a person you don't really love. A relationship that is nothing more than an accommodation of our insecurities is a dangerous path to embark upon. Unfortunately this is an all too common problem, and children in particular suffer from our mistakes. The proof is in studies showing 55 percent of all marriages in this country ending in divorce, and many still-married spouses saying they would have already separated or divorced if they could afford it.

How is it possible that our society can have such a high failure rate in satisfying relationships? One fundamental reason is that so many people get into serious relationships before they have developed an authentic relationship with themselves. How can we contain so much insecurity, uncertainty, dysfunction, fear, and sense of incompletion and expect something healthy and authentic to come forth? Living an inauthentic life, conditioned by the negative moments from our past, makes us hide our foibles. We are afraid to be identified with our weaknesses and failures so we compensate by wearing masks and putting on airs. We give the appearance of being secure, happy, responsible, conscientious, and industrious. But then where is the real person? When our masks are removed we are simply human beings existing on the edge of a void, busying ourselves running around the edges of darkness so we don't have to realize we are already in it. With our social commitments and careers, life turns into a huge effort in multitasking. If we have kids too, there is even less time left to examine anything meaningful about ourselves. You pass your significant other in the house and forget who each other is. We are trying to do so many things that we can hardly do even one thing well. If you don't give quality time to anything you do, everything will eventually suffer. It's like making an electrical repair in the home; you can either do it properly or you can mend it temporarily. In American society we are masters of temporary repairs, such as temporary healthcare, temporary commissions that discuss problems without providing sustainable resolutions, and temporary measures in New Orleans after Hurricane Katrina. Little is done authentically and therefore few problems are actually solved.

So what kind of life are you living if it is not a sustainable life? Whenever I am confronted by a choice, I have to decide whether it can be sustained in a complete and balanced way; if it can't, then I should not do it. Moreover, everything in life, every choice, is an exchange. If I am going to exchange imbalance for balance, then I must surrender everything that generates imbalance. Wasting time creates imbalance. Giving our energy to pursuits that are trivial and undeserving of our effort creates instability. Absorbing the energy of other people who are not constructive and positive in turn imbalances us. Living in a toxic environment upsets our lives. When we are imbalanced, unhealthy, and caught in a web of inauthentic relationships, everything we undertake is going to be based on a fear of losing whatever it is we feel a need to control. When we exert a lot of energy by trying to control something we feel we are losing a handle on we imbalance ourselves further. For example, people try to control others with jealousy. Jealousy is a straightjacket we wrap around someone else, but it immobilizes us simultaneously. How comfortable are we with ourselves and with another person when we are in a straightjacket together?

Envy is another form of control. We see a person with something we don't have and we feel incomplete without it, so we try to get it for ourselves. When we finally acquire the object of our envy we realize we were better off without it. All we really received for our efforts are bills: an emotional bill, a time-wasted bill, and a misused energy bill.

Take a glance at all of the things you own and once felt you needed but never really had a use for—they're a concrete example of decisions that originated from a place of imbalance. Fear, insecurity, the lack of an authentic sense of self, the feeling of an incomplete life, and giving up positive for negative energy all create imbalance. A common phrase we hear from people's lips is "I wish it were Friday." That is actually a terrible thought because it means today doesn't count. It suggests that there is little real life and little real sacredness in today. Moreover, underlying this thought is the false assurance that if you get through today then tomorrow will be better. This is simply a negative exchange of energy: an exchange of the reality of this moment for the illusion that tomorrow is going to be a better moment. And how often does tomorrow turn out to be any better? Instead we should be asking about what we need in order to create balance. Once there is balance, there is less disease and disharmony.

How often do you find yourself obsessing over something that didn't go the way you had expected? Afterwards you find yourself rerunning a parade of thoughts to death. "Well, I should have said this," or, "I should have done that." You repeat those mantras over and over in your mind. How does thinking obsessively about something that happened in the past change anything? It doesn't. You just surrendered precious time to obsess over it. You exchanged an opportunity to let it go for an opportunity to engage your mind in reliving compulsive thoughts. You need to surrender what you cannot control, and should not control, and simply be present to accept the moment you are in. From there you can see clearly the choices that will guide you positively.

So be conscious and be present. Surrender everything that imbalances you and replace it with something that creates an authentic, sustainable life. Love, joy, hopefulness, vulnerability, and a pure belief in yourself are qualitative energies of an authentic life. When you connect to those energies you support your growth, surrendering all of your past conditioned needs that no longer fit into your life and replacing them with the sense of your real self in this moment. When you do that you are ready for remarkable moments because you are open and vulnerable to experience them. The reason why every day is not a remarkable moment is because we are carrying yesterday into today in order to justify the way we feel. We repeat old behavioral patterns over and over as if our behaviors will miraculously produce different results. We should stop fighting yesterday's battles.

Fear is perhaps the single most important motivating factor locking us down into an inauthentic, artificial life, which curtails much of our potential for growth. We construct our existence out of the building blocks of our fears. Certainly we all go through the motions of making efforts, believing we are changing because we have different experiences—relationships, different jobs and residences, a variety of interests and activities. However, experiences aren't truly relevant unless we treat them as lessons and grow during the process of facing them. And the lesson of fear is one of the most important lessons to confront.

One way to deal with your fears is by consciously experimenting with your life and beliefs. If we are afraid of connecting with and expressing our honesty, some of what we say and do is based on fear. Some conversations can't be authentic because the conversation aims to be accepted and to avoid criticism and rejection. So for one full day, commit yourself to being completely honest about everything you say and think. Detach yourself from all your fears about imagined consequences and just be honest and allow events to unfold. There is no need to be mean, cruel, or harsh in your words and tone. Simply be compassionate and honest but also uncompromising and see what happens. Speak gently and truthfully to everyone you talk to and observe the responses you receive.

When we are absolutely honest with ourselves, we are raising the standards by which we feel, act, and communicate with others. Living an honest life enables new and remarkable events to unfold for us. We discover that the rewards gained for being honest are far greater than those when we were entangled in our inauthentic, conditioned self.

During conversations, listen attentively without the conditioned ego's prejudgment. Only then will you be able to respond honestly because your authentic self will be processing the information. Instead of personalizing your conversations, go into neutral. Whenever you personalize, you become upset with whatever disagrees with your feelings and your needs. The subconscious mind activates when you are upset and launches a volley of conditioned responses, which may result in your reacting from your ego. The ego will try to subordinate the real self because it is the master of all your defense mechanisms. Why do you think so few people won't attempt to undertake anything out of the cultural norm? It is because their defense mechanisms defend and justify their fears. The ego circumvents authentic risk-taking that will lead to growth and illumination. It is important to understand that if people denigrate your inspiration, they are not really listening; they are reacting, not toward you, but toward themselves. Their egos, not their authentic selves, are conditioned to react. The ego serves as the frontline attack dog for every belief system, reacting on impulse because that is how the ego is hard-wired to respond throughout a person's life. By surrendering the ego, we surrender fear as well. Only after the ego is under control does the authentic self speak, hear, and feel.

If you wish to appreciate the meaning of enlightenment, this wonderful sense of illumination, it is important to understand the transcendental state of consciousness. In a transcendental state, you surrender your sense of a personal "I" and connect instead with the sense of "we." In this state you achieve a conscious connection with the entire world. You are present with everyone all races, ethnicities, ages, and ideas. There is no need to force your ideas on anyone, nor is there a tendency to personalize whatever is being shared with you. Behind every religion, every ideological belief, every cultural and political difference, there are simply human beings. When you surrender your need to define yourself through your ego with all of its cultural conditionings and let go your need to be right, you discover yourself aligned with the correctness of the universe. The universe offers a far more extraordinary connection than anything you could discover when being unconsciously led by the ego.

So many of us have become master artisans of believing that we are all that matters in the world. We build our homes hedged and fenced away from our neighbors and don't bother to barter and exchange. We may resent the successes of others and fear our own losses. And what do we fear most? The loss of our youth, of our money and success, of our popularity, and of our relationships and security. Anyone who has the need to seek their way into the higher citadels of power will most fear the loss of that power and control. We cling to all of these illusions even though they are fleeting at best. We all know deep inside that some parts of the life we live are illusions. But the authentic self is constantly open to universal truth. Every cell in our bodies contains universal truth, which our minds and bodies can connect with at any moment. This truth is not simply the "I" we have all come to believe as the center of the universe. It is the "we" of all life that really matters and is most real.

What do we all have in common? When we hear someone say, "You and I have a lot in common," the first thing that comes to mind is mutual interests, hobbies, lifestyles, music and movies, social status, or educational background. These are all constructs glossing over the more important commonality everyone on the planet shares: we are all human beings with an innate desire to be happy, honored, respected, and appreciated; in other words, a need for true intimacy. When we fail to meet another person as a human being we get caught up in labels that either draw us closer together or push us further apart. When we label a person by race, religion, ethnicity, political and economic orientation, or education, we are raising the stature of these differences above what is real and true. But these distinctions make no difference because none of them are essential. On the other hand, when we meet someone as a human being, with the motivation to honor each other's experience, an authentic connection is made. This is how two people meet at a transcendental level. This is how peace and love are generated. This is how war and violence are brought to an end.

Every cell in your body is aware at the transcendental level until you superimpose your ego's will and thought upon your body and mind. If your ego says you are no good and unworthy, then you will be bad and unworthy. If the ego doubts you can do something you will never do it. The way we identify and associate with an authority figure and a ruling paradigm will also control our perceptions about ourselves and determine our ability to express our freedom to choose and act. So for a moment, step back and consider a question. What if the many limiting things you've been told are wrong? What if you are really deep down a good, smart human being who wants to think and live independently and creatively?

Every day is a new opportunity to reexamine how we can make our life better and richer with remarkable experiences. Now you can make the rest of your days remarkable; you can become open to the transcendental process, whether through meditation, quiet moments, contemplative presence in nature, journaling, a personal breakdown or catharsis, or a spontaneous epiphany. The way in which you transcend depends upon your circumstances, but you must open yourself fearlessly to discover that every day is remarkable. When you reside in the illuminated state of mind, living itself is an experience of grace. This is the state of illumination.

CHAPTER FIVE

Expanding into Enlightenment

There is an old story from India that serves as an excellent tool for understanding the meaning of our expanding into enlightenment. The story was made popular in the 1800s by John Godfrey Saxe in his poem entitled "The Blind Men and the Elephant." Once there was a group of blind wise men who sought out an elephant to try to understand its nature. One wise man grabbed the trunk and said it was a snake. Another felt the animal's ear and mistook it for a fan. The tusk felt like a spear. The elephant's frame was a wall, the leg a tree, and the tail a rope. None of the wise men were correct, yet each believed he was right. Saxe's poem reveals how the personal truths we live by seduce us into mistaking a part of a problem for the entire reality.

When we grope through life with our eyes closed, we may wake up one morning and think, *My God, here's my to-do list and I'm not even on it! I can't handle all these tasks when I should be dealing with my everyday relationships and responsibilities, my self-image, my children and community.* We usually panic at this point and use various coping mechanisms to numb out. Some people will buy things they don't need, or overeat, or watch too much TV. Others go gambling; or they first take tranquilizers and then go gambling so they won't feel bad after they lose. We distract ourselves and we find numerous targets to blame for our troubles: society, our childhood, a boss, abuse, or neglect. But we give little thought to the choices we make that are the true cause of our problems. Do you see the endless games we play?

So how can we bring clarity, some enlightening awareness, to our problems and lives? How can we rediscover joy and happiness and gain mastery over ourselves and our environment?

First, you need to thoroughly clean up the mess you find yourself living in. Rearranging the parts of a large problem does not solve anything. Everything in your life needs to be changed so you can start anew. A fresh start is only possible after you recognize that something you are clinging to needs to be surrendered. Two different energies cannot share the same space with equal intensity at the same time. If you're holding onto something negative, you cannot hold on to a positive energy and expect something good and healthy to manifest for you simultaneously. There are many things you can do to start changing your life. To begin this process, I will set forth some lessons for you to follow. Adhering to the exact order as I present them is not necessary: you can change the order as it best suits you. If you are starting at a point where you are out of balance, the first thing to do is learn to step back. If you are ill, overweight, anxious, angry, or depressed there is a lack of balance. And the first way to correct this is to step back and ask, *Where am I out of balance? Where am I putting my energy?*

One reason why people are so frustrated and accumulate negative energy leading to disease and suffering is because they cannot control others or get what they want. How many things in life can you actually control? The only thing you can exert real control over is how you choose to feel about yourself and the world. When we can't control or possess our desires, we tend to resort to force, which by its very nature is a negative energy.

Everything in life is energy: every feeling, every experience, and every location. There are two principle energies in life: the positive and the negative. Positive energy is a very light energy. Why do we feel content gazing at the ocean or sitting quietly by a lake? Why do we experience joy in the presence of children, pets, and positive people? It is because the energy they are sharing with us is positive. How often do we take a little bit of that energy as a respite and fall right back into the negative vortex when we return to work, our family, or friends? So many people say to themselves, *Well, I feel secure with my job and money is coming in. There are people who I consider friends and who understand me. What else do I need?* Yet their lives remain toxic. They are willing to exchange true happiness and an authentic life for a superficial security, which is imbalanced. Others are convinced that redemption comes from their suffering, but we are not a better person if we suffer. We are merely a more toxic person.

Do you see where this is leading? First we need to look at the nature of disease and unhappiness and how it is related to the wrong choices we make. Our wrong choices happen when there is a lack of balance. If you are not in balance with your body it is going to get sick. But if you make a real effort to pay attention—manifest only positive energy, eat the right foods and nutrients, commit to right thoughts and right actions—you can rebalance your body. And the only way to rebalance your body is to first rebalance your mind. How is the mind rebalanced? By putting a halt to conflict. When conflict is absent, greater clarity is available to us. When the mind is balanced, all decisions become less difficult because in true enlightenment there is a sense of ease. There is no need to control the outcome of our decisions.

Insecurity and fear so often prevent us from making positive exchanges, but there is an exercise we can all do, a simple practice that can have a profound impact on changing our lives for the better. Visualize what you need and then project your visualized need into the universe. Just take your thought and put it out there. Now here's the key: don't chase your need. Don't force it or try to control or manipulate it. Just let it go out into the universe without any effort. As I mentioned, everything in life is energy: every rock, plant, animal, and person. Everything vibrates; it's all alive. So if I believe in the interconnection and completeness of life, when I put out a need, I'm also trusting that the universe understands. Every time I've had a situation when I needed something and I put that energy out into the universe, and worked on it with discipline, focus, and patience, I have received what I asked for. People will argue these are just coincidences, but when you have done this enough and experienced the results, you will think very differently.

All energy is cumulative. People don't just wake up overweight one morning, but over time; people rarely become bankrupt immediately, but through mounting debt. Relationships are not destroyed the day after partners fall in love. There are other negative energies involved that are cumulative. Our lowest points in life are reached when one day we have exchanged so many positive things for negative ones that our balance is completely lost. And so often that tipping point manifests as a disease in the body, such as a heart attack, stroke, or cancer. But it was all cumulative. It may have taken twenty or thirty years for the disease to progress to the appearance of symptoms; just because you don't observe evident symptoms doesn't mean you are not manifesting a negative energy that is an actual disease in process. You may not have lung cancer from smoking today or a damaged liver from drinking when you wake up tomorrow. But sooner or later the accumulation of negative energy—in your thoughts, behavior, and environment—will take its toll.

So on that day when you finally say, "My God, I don't know why I am so sick," take a look at the accumulation of all your beliefs and actions, of cause and effect, and you will discover that your situation reflects your actions, which always follow your beliefs. Realize that you have become whatever your mind told you. Our beliefs are only perceptions, and our perceptions are defined and controlled by the particular paradigm we buy into. The next step for learning to exchange energy positively is to reflect on what is necessary to live a sustainable life. If we begin to live every day with the idea of sustainable living, then we will only make choices that we can realistically sustain. Say I want to sustain my health. Then what do I have to do? Well, I need to make different choices around food and exercise, exchanging my negative habits and thoughts for positive ones. How do I sustain my happiness? I need to be around people who are internally joyful and, whenever possible, avoid dysfunctional people. We feel weighted down in the presence of people who hold onto the negative energy of unhappiness. How many times have you found yourself acting as a rescuer, only to discover the person crying to be rescued has wrapped a rope around your waist with a giant boulder and is leaping off a cliff? You can't rescue people; ultimately they have to want to be rescued. A person who demands to be rescued may be manipulating a game that you do not understand. They've mastered it and they will take your energy down to the dark recesses where they reside as victims.

When you see how our society connects with that which is negative, it informs you about what we have become as a culture and as a nation. You can begin to understand the dynamics behind why people gamble, smoke, drink, and pursue negative activities with destructive results. And it will come as no surprise how popular our media's moronic shock jocks are, and why they are rewarded with multimillion dollar contracts while Nobel Peace Prize winners toil in relative obscurity. What does this tell us? It tells us we are collectively living at the negative end of the energy spectrum.

When we feel a need to belong and act on that need, we exchange our sense of autonomy, our authentic self-image, for something that doesn't put positive energy out in the universe. We lose our ability to appreciate who we truly are. But you can put the positive energy for sustainable needs out there and wait for it to return. It will come back, so be patient. When the energy does return, you'll be connecting with what is really authentic and meaningful for living a healthy, enlightened life.

In order to unclutter and simplify our lives, we must surrender what we no longer desire to be. This allows the energy of our authentic selves to emerge. But as long as we're holding onto one energy a different energy cannot take its place. That's why we tend to think at higher levels and act on lower impulses. We think light but act heavy; we think spiritually but act nonspiritually. We think positively but act negatively. We keep exchanging the energy for what we ideally want because we're not willing to surrender the energy we have become. Let's say you and your partner plan to have a future together, a simple life where you can both do all the things you've always wanted. But it's going to be rough reaching that goal: seventeen-hour work days, less time spent together, nights of exhaustion, and no end in sight. Yet that is all right because the paradigm tells us we are supposed to get married, have children, buy a home, overwork, create debt, stress ourselves, and make superficial friends. The paradigm tells us security is to be found by closing our eyes like the blind men and tolerating the illusion. This is how people go along living and then wake up one day and realize they're overweight, alcoholic, or seriously ill—they have been sublimating from the frustration of not living an authentic life.

Our most important lesson is to learn to be present in this moment. When I'm in this moment and I'm conscious of this moment, my conscious focus allows me to make any choice I want with utmost clarity. I can exchange any negative energy for any positive one. Then I can put my feelings into the universe and know they are honest and authentic ones. I can observe things and situations for what they are. Conditioned responses no longer exist in this moment because I see everything, hear everything, clearly. I don't need to vet, interpret, or edit my clarity through any belief system.

Our belief systems cause us to take things out of context, which is how we are able to continue justifying violence, racism, sexism, and our personal dysfunctions. Whenever we exchange truth for an illusion, we are permitting ourselves to continue stoking the fire of our passions to think and act in negative ways. But in the present moment, there is only clarity. In the moment of clarity you have authentic control over yourself and can surrender illusion. This is where we gain enlightenment, because in this moment you can choose to make authentic choices. Enlightenment in life is fundamentally about the quality of the choices we make and our willingness to stand behind them.

We tend to lose touch with those moments of enlightenment when we fall into our routines. It's possible to be awake and alive to the present moment amidst routine, but usually we go on autopilot with repetition. Routines are a continuation of past rituals, habits, and patterns: eating the same diet, dressing the same way, watching the same television programs, taking the same medications. Most people pride themselves in regimenting themselves with their routines. They don't break their habits or challenge them. They don't surrender them in exchange for something better. We have to examine and change our routines to see where we are actually at.

One way to live at an enlightened level is by engaging in what I call *conscious creating*. You do this by starting to create wonderful ideas while being conscious in the moment. Avoid the habit of convincing yourself you do not have enough money or you are not educated enough. All you have to do is trust that the universe will help you create an idea and you suddenly find the energy starts to lighten up. Creative energy is a rapid, vibrating energy. Try to be creative with everything you do, in every area of your life. Have fun with it. Play with the energy. If you're not creating then your energy stagnates, and stagnant energy is negative energy. It drains you. The less you create, the less positive energy you have at your disposal. The more you create, the lighter your energy becomes.

At the end of the day, it is really a simple, uncomplicated pleasant life that we all deserve and yearn for. But our choices often remove us from our ideal life. The place we live can take it away. Our jobs can, too. Even our friends and associates can remove us from what we need most. Instead of moving closer to our ideal, we remain in our ideal's antithesis. This generates such anxiety, depression, and apathy that we find ourselves succumbing to drinking, smoking, overeating, or taking medications to vent our sense of incompleteness. So we must work at rebalancing ourselves and simplifying our lives to feel that we are sufficient as we are every day, and discover the enlightenment possible in each moment.

CHAPTER SIX

The Thirteenth Step

Today in America, tens of millions of individuals suffer from one or more kinds of addictive behavior. There are now approximately one hundred and forty million overweight Americans, over fifty million people who continue to smoke, and over two hundred million who display symptoms of sugar craving. Add to these figures the millions of others who gamble, consume alcohol and coffee, or are chronic workaholics, and you begin to realize the vast condition of suffering spreading throughout this nation.

In this chapter I will outline a program called the Thirteenth Step to help combat the rampant addictions so many of us struggle with. It is a method of self-empowerment that will enable you to gain greater mastery over yourself and your life choices in order to live a happier and healthier life. Why do I offer a Thirteenth Step when we already have twelve-step programs, which have clearly benefited countless people? Based upon my own experience with my extended family, who have struggled with various addictions, it seemed that some fundamental understanding was still lacking. Despite my family members' sincere attempts to rebalance their lives, more often than not their efforts turned futile.

In a halfway house in Florida, a group of people I know struggles to recover from their dysfunctions and return to society. The house members have either been in jail, been victims of traumatic marriages, or lost their means of livelihood. They have identified themselves as alcoholics, addicts, or chronic gamblers. Their greatest wish is to live a life that brings them joy and happiness. During my time getting to know these people, I started to realize that even in the absence of a particular addiction or dysfunctional behavior, a person will not necessarily be happy or healthy.

How often have you heard someone say, "Well, I no longer drink alcohol," but he or she continues to drink coffee, smokes, or consumes lots of sugar? At an AA meeting I attended with one of my family members, I watched participants smoking cigarettes, drinking coffee, and devouring sweets before and after the session. I realized that underneath the surface of coping with their many habits, they were full of anger or rage. So it is important that these recovery programs provide the spiritual component of recovery that they do, but there are still pieces of the puzzle that are missing. The program I am presenting will look at recovery differently, more holistically.

From the outset, I want it understood that I do not believe that anyone has an addiction disease. By being quick to label problems a disease, the medical establishment pathologizes symptoms that have a deeper, more essential cause. How many times do we hear and read that alcoholism is a disease; and now medicine has defined being overweight as a disease too. But what if unhealthy weight gain and addictive behavior such as drinking and smoking, gambling, shopping, and overeating are illnesses of the mind and spirit? Then there are no real medications for treatment.

Each of us must begin by asking ourselves a series of questions in order to embark upon a new mode of thinking about ourselves and the world around us. We will each discover our own unique answers;

the questions I offer are merely suggestions to initiate this new thinking process.

Let's look at one essential human quality that is frequently absent from our lives: happiness. I do not mean the fleeting feeling of pleasure, but rather the happiness that can be experienced and sustained in a balanced relationship between the body, mind, and spirit. For a moment, reflect upon how we reinforce our loss of self by neglecting our happiness before we hit a time of crisis; the loss of a job, a serious illness, the passing of a loved one. When we neglect our emotional, intellectual, and creative growth during times of relative stability, we are unconsciously increasing the magnitude of our loss when a crisis appears.

How many people across the cities and towns of America wake every morning and spend their days working in an environment that does not honor them? They fall into a routine to pay the rent or mortgage. Their apartments and homes turn into little more than way stations, points of transition empty of warmth and real comfort, as they work to keep up with paying bills. More often than not, people are too exhausted from their careers and routines to enjoy even the inexpensive and free places that bring vitality and beauty to life: botanical gardens, a zoo, museums and galleries, strolls in parks and nature. Instead they postpone their lives, waiting for "when I get financially secure," "when I find the right relationship," or "when I feel good enough or get my health back." But all they are doing is putting their life on hold until something outside themselves is achieved, believing that only then will they live the life they are meant to live. We make our possessions more valuable than they deserve; we have charged them with emotional significance. But our lives are far more significant than any thing we can own.

I know many people who earn a lot of money, but it's still not enough for them to create a schedule that gives them freedom to experience life's fullness. One of the most humbling experiences we can have is realizing that the world will go on without any of us. Underneath the stress and anxiety that gnaws away at us is the profound sense of our life's impermanence: the impermanence of our youth, our body, our relationships, and our culture.

How do we react when we are stressed and helpless to change the conditions bearing down on us? We sublimate. We sublimate when we can't cope with something in our lives, such as a situation we can't correct or a confrontation that disempowers us. When we are faced with these situations, we sublimate by overeating, shopping, or using alcohol and drugs, keeping ourselves busy in order to evade our deeper problems. Addictive habits are not the real problem, but merely symptoms. Because most self-improvement programs focus on the symptoms as fundamental problems, we miss seeing the deeper imbalances that drive us. If you can identify what is imbalanced in yourself, you will discover the cause of stress leading to your feeling of helplessness, and consequently the reasons for dealing with problems improperly. So the symptoms are not a disease or a pathology but the result of inappropriate behavior, of making wrong choices.

How many times in your life have you reflected on the past and questioned the choices you made or could have made? We've all thought many times, *If only I had not said what I said, things would be different*. But it was done and it can't be changed. What we can do is not repeat those same mistakes. We can learn from them and realize how our inappropriate choices created imbalance in our life. If we decide to hide something in a relationship, what are we going to receive in return? Whatever it is we fear most. If you fear abandonment, then you may be abandoned.

So we need to embrace the problem. The problem is not outside us; it is not about who we have hurt, or about who hurt us. The underlying cause of the problem is wrong choices, which can build into crises. In most cases we choose our own crises. We refuse to acknowledge this because it requires taking responsibility and being accountable for the results. What happens when we do take responsibility for a situation gone awry? Yes, we may feel some guilt or shame, but we will also feel relief from having been honest and can understand the decisions that don't contribute to our happiness and goals in life. So pay attention to those crucial questions about where you want to be, what you truly want in life, and how you want to feel about yourself. That's where you should concentrate your energy. The answer to these questions is where you will find balance in your life.

It's important to understand that if you haven't found what you need it's because you're not looking in the right places. How many times have you become angry or apologetic and then declared you will never repeat that mistake or make that wrong decision again, and then you end up doing it again anyway? You can cry all you want, can confess all you want, but that's no guarantee that anything will change for the better. Because if you never release, never surrender your anger and resentments, you will never touch your deeper self.

When an opportunity arises to make a change and try something new, we so often stop in our tracks and refrain from taking advantage of the opportunity. Beneath our hesitation is a deep fear about what is unpredictable if we become our real self. We are fearful of where an important change will lead us. When we go to a deeper level of the self, we are identifying with our true authenticity as a human being.

So many people are rigid and closed toward all that is unfamiliar to them and react to the unknown with fear and trepidation. You can't give unconditional love to others until you love yourself. This is why so few people are authentically loving and open to strangers and to the world. If I feel unconditional love, and if I can stay present with that unconditional love in this moment, then I can't judge other people. I look at others and everything around me with love instead of with critical disdain. Now imagine what would happen if people who were in a crisis looked at each other with love instead of hate. When you look at people with love, even those who have hurt or denied you, you see in them the same things that you want to see in yourself and can realize that everyone who has ever committed a bad act can also do something very good.

When crisis is absent from our lives, what should we be paying attention to? Are there changes still to be made, and if so, what are they? In most cases, people do nothing when their lives are crisis-free because safety is found in predictable patterns, in clinging to the same habits.

One of the fundamental reasons why we resist change is because we fear our resources for managing the consequences are limited or unavailable. Most often this translates into feeling that we simply do not have the capability to undertake a major change. This pattern of thinking turns increasingly into an ingrained habit as we grow older. When opportunities arise to make a concerted change in our lives, we always have excuses: not enough money, insufficient knowledge, not having the right connections.

Frequently we focus on what we don't want. But that gives those things power. There are days when we are engaged in the very thing we didn't want. Your choice of thought creates both positive and negative outcomes. When stability and security are valued above everything else, there can be no positive change. Everything you do will be grounded in a false sense of security.

What benefit is there in facing your crisis, and what happens when you embrace it? You become responsible. You own your failure and realize the act of confronting your crisis in some cases is more important than the crisis itself. Most people do not learn this lesson. They enter an electric storm with thunder and lightning, are pelted by heavy rain, and think, *Wait a minute! I hate this. I better take cover.* So they hunker down and insulate themselves because the storm overwhelms them. But suppose you make the decision to keep moving forward through the storm, and you witness a magnificent rainbow on the other side? The rainbow is the moment of enlightenment behind the crisis' message for you. The message is what redeems the crisis.

If you learn the lesson of a crisis by embracing it, then you will be less likely to repeat it. Then you are free. You are free not only from alcohol, drugs, overeating, gambling, and shopping but from your deeper need to make improper choices to cover up anxiety and stress. You become grounded; you're fully awake and present in the moment.

When people gain weight, go bankrupt, or succumb to self-destructive addictions, they often experience shame and embarrassment, and they are left with the feeling of having failed. Whose company do they tend to seek and attract when they feel like failures? Frequently other people who feel like failures. Instead, we should be seeking the company of people who are healthy role models—happy, vital, and positive about their lives.

Self-improvement programs should begin by affirming in participants that they are human beings—not alcoholics, addicts, or overweight. You are just a human being who made inappropriate choices, so the question is, what is the lesson to be learned from your crisis? Where is your rainbow? If you understand the deeper cause of your crisis, the next time you will not feel helpless, and you won't revert to making inappropriate choices again. Otherwise, you might not overeat or drink anymore, but no progress, no true self-realization, is gained if you return home and hit your spouse or kick the cat. Eighty percent of people going through recovery wind up back where they started. Only when you surrender your anger and give up your insecurity and codependency do you start to make real progress. Otherwise, you can stand up in meetings and confess all you want with a momentary relief that you have redeemed yourself, but nothing substantial will change. If you continue to believe you are fighting a demon every second of every day, always putting on your mental armor, your mindset can project the energy into the universe that you "fear relapse," so the universe gives you back "relapse energy." Change the mindset. Yes, you made wrong choices, but you learned what choices you could and will make. Lesson learned; go on with your life.

We learn some of life's greatest lessons by associating with people who are happy, joyful, and loving, who make proper choices in life, in contrast to most of us who focus on just making it through the next twenty-four hours. If you are only striving to make it through the next day without any sense of joy or purpose, you have hit a barrier that hinders progress and growth. You might make it through a day without having a drink or eating a box of chocolates, but you continue to feel the weight of stress. You may have not indulged yourself, but you still feel rage. Instead say, *I'm just a human being and it's going to be a beautiful day for me. I'm going to focus only on what I need to do to make the right choices.*

People usually reach a point in their lives where it is too much hassle to start something over again with a new perspective. It is easier and safer to adapt to the image of ourselves we are most comfortable with. It may not be the best relationship or the ideal job, but it is paying the bills and sustains a certain standard of living. However, whenever we adapt to something negative our lives will be thrown out of balance by our compromises.

Compromise does not always achieve anything positive. Sometimes we compromise when we don't take the time to consider a better alternative. Some compromises generate imbalance; imbalance creates conflict, leading to more serious crises. Only then do we realize we have developed a debilitating disease, are in a codependent relationship, or waste four precious hours a day commuting to work. We compromise ourselves and adapt to situations when we feel we can't change them. As you transform your crisis you will discover a new relationship to your experience, and the cause of your difficulties will become crystal clear. Only when you connect with what is authentic and true can you identify with the authenticity of your own existence. When you do that, you can make constructive changes. So it is exceedingly important to reflect on what is authentic in yourself because this is where the answers for finding balance reside. Everything that is not authentic leads to imbalance. Frustrations, anger, stress, and disappointment always have their roots in what is not authentic.

Why do you think so many people who appear remarkably successful are also self-destructive? What is lacking? They do not have an authentic sense of self. They are not present to the fullness of their life. Their apparent success is no more than a shadow chasing after them. Underneath the surface, they reside in a dark, damp basement piled high with depression and hopelessness, without windows allowing the light of happiness and completeness to enter. It is easy and comfortable to reside in the shadow of who we should be while continuing to make inappropriate choices, but those choices will inevitably burst into a crisis.

Investigate where there is distortion in your life. Anything that's distorted needs to be faced and corrected. One way of removing distortions from life is by correcting the illusory image of what you imagine you ought to be. For example, many of us hold an illusion about what happiness, or a great job, or a loving relationship should be. Yet if that image were to manifest it would neither be happy nor loving. The result is disappointment and a sense of failure. We then find consolation in watching TV and movies, reading inane novels, believing that new perfected images will be found there. Disillusioned with our lives, we become enamored by the lives of others. When we sink into our own illusions, our lives become smaller and we believe our options lessen. We have very little appreciation for the uniqueness of our being. We are always raising somebody or something to a higher pedestal. This is just one more illusion in our world full of illusions. Unconsciously we often live constricted, limited lives, but this is not our authentic self.

How do you respond when an unforeseeable event forces you to interrupt your routine behavior? For example, you are in a routine of doing something daily, but then something disrupts your routine. In most cases, you react with anger, fear, depression, or anxiety. The reason is that you were unprepared. The disruption presented you with a situation you were unable to cope with, and you plunged yourself into what you knew was safe and secure: becoming stressed or depressed, overeating, or using alcohol or drugs. Instead, if anything disrupts your normal routine, you should acknowledge that it may not be pleasant and is not what you had hoped for, but it awakens your attention and that in itself is valuable. Our normal routines and behavior are not conducive to keeping a clear awareness.

On the other hand, disruptions and crises force us to pay more attention.

So what must we do when our routines change suddenly? We need to remain in the present moment, become detached and neutral, let the change unfold, and pay attention to it. Look at a change or deeper crisis as an opportunity and ask, *How do I want to respond to this?*

When you remove all the illusions you cling to and come face-to-face with the bare truth of who you really are, that's the moment when your journey begins. You may not be thrilled with the timing of this encounter or with the commitment demanded of you, but when you are forced to be brutally honest with yourself, you are creating a new foundation for your life that is on solid ground. There are no more lies or deceptions about who you are. Everything you build on this foundation will help you to evolve. When your foundation is based upon truth and authenticity, you can evolve in unlimited ways.

So rid yourself of the illusion you have been living and realize the truth: your mistakes in the past, your poor choices, are not the real you. Because you were ill-prepared to deal with a crisis or a crucial challenge, you made inappropriate decisions. There is no reason to beat yourself up or become angry or depressed over the past; you simply did not have the right tools.

We grow up on the day that we realize we are an extension of all the mistakes we have made. So forgive yourself for making those wrong choices, and forgive other people who made wrong choices concerning you. Forgive all the institutions, which in their ignorance deceived you with falsehoods. Forgive everything in your life that has played a part in creating the illusion that you've become. Then look at who you really are, the authentic, true you. If no one else accepts you for who you truly are, at least you accept yourself. That is all you need because, in the end, you are born alone and will die alone. There is no need to try to prove yourself to other people. We frustrate ourselves when we try to prove to others that we are deserving of their attention, love, kindness, and respect. This is when we start compromising and adapting to our illusory patterns of ourselves. Instead simply say, *This is who I am. Like me and respect me because I know myself. I honor myself and everyone else.*

With this acceptance of yourself and others, conflict can dissolve and you can be in balance. Where there's balance, there's harmony. And where there's harmony, there is bliss. In bliss, there's no need to sublimate. When you're not sublimating, then there's no destructive behavior leading to addictions. You will understand that addictions are not diseases because you have discovered the root cause of your struggles and found freedom in your new awareness.

CHAPTER SEVEN

Attracting Success through Self-Empowerment

I believe it is possible to succeed at almost everything in life. I also believe we don't tend to give enough attention to understanding how to achieve this success and examine the ways we ourselves are the primary cause for our lives unfolding the way they do. To understand how and why success manifests in our lives, we must look at a principle called *attracting success*. Imagine that we are magnets or magnetized energy. When any thought—positive or negative—is sent out into the universe, the universe responds and returns the thought back to us. If we have prepared ourselves to receive whatever we have asked for, the universe responds to our request and we become more successful. So through this unity of request and response, we can have everything we want: health, happiness, joy, an expansion of consciousness, and clear awareness.

However, there is a caveat to this concept of attracting what we need: Everything that we do not want, yet continue to exert our thoughts toward, the universe will also provide. In fact, this is what most often happens because we entertain more thoughts about what we don't want than about what we do. How often do we hear, "I don't want to be lied to," or "I don't want to be cheated or manipulated," or "I don't want to be broke and owe more bills." But these negative wants are exactly what we will end up manifesting because we have fed what we don't want with so much energy.

I am going to offer some practical steps to stimulate you to think differently. Interpret them as they best suit you. Ultimately you are the architect, the designer of the answer; I merely frame the questions. We cannot change the patterns and ways our lives unfold if we remain in the same mindset and hold the same energy that has brought us to the point we find ourselves in now. If a person is rich, powerful, and famous but still feels empty, frustrated, and lonely, making more money and achieving more success will not bring him or her any closer to a satisfying sense of a fulfilled life. So what can you do to make the principle of energy exchange a positive force in your life? First you need to decide what you really want to do. Then focus on that with clear intention to the exclusion of everything else. Our culture takes pride in a person's ability to multitask, but you should perform only one exercise at a time, with one intention at a time. Never focus on what you don't want; only on what you do want. If you focus yourself, meditate, and then send your intention into the universe, it will return to you.

However, a couple of questions still remain. First, are you prepared to receive the energy you have requested or are you still blocked? In other words, even though you have the desire to receive something, are you capable of actualizing it when it does return to you? Many people dream and fantasize about being more complete and more wholesome in their lives, but they have yet to surrender their negative energies to allow new positive energies a place to anchor. They continue to vibrate with insecurity, fear, anger, and irrational thoughts, reactionary energies they have mastered from their past. We have all mastered negative energy; now it's time to learn mastery of positive energy instead.

Because no two opposite energies are capable of sharing the same space at the same time, the degree to which you can surrender everything that holds you back is the degree that you can open yourself to grow. Otherwise, even though you want something very positive, you will not be ready to accept it. Very often fear prevents us from being prepared, so it is crucial to overcome fear, surrendering the energy associated with memories that condition you to be fearful. A very helpful exercise is to make a list of everything you want to rid yourself of and then focus on each thing's positive manifestation. For example, if I do not want to be fat, then I focus only on what it means to be thinner. If I do not want to be sick, then I should focus on what it means to be well. If I no longer want to feel depressed, I have to make an effort to focus on feeling happy. If I am angry at people and want to rid myself of hostile thoughts, I need to focus on loving others. So always focus on the positive aspect of what you want to remove, and master that positive energy. Then that new energy will vibrate, and like a magnet you will attract the positive thoughts and needs you put out into the universe. Otherwise, if you feel doubtful, you will continue to attract doubting people or if you are always angry, you will continue to meet other angry people. We can observe every day how easily negative people bond with each other due to their similar vibrations.

We can actualize and materialize our needs through visualization. Before we practice visualization, first we need to find some quality time to quiet the mind. Our lives are usually so cluttered that we cannot properly focus. We unclutter our situation by identifying what we no longer want in our lives and then, with concerted intention, take back the time these things occupy in our everyday routines. It might mean removing the TV, radio, or newspapers, or not engaging in meaningless conversations. When you do that, you will be amazed at how many extra hours you will free up in your day for more meaningful activity.

When we are living in the proper location, doing the right work, acting with the right attitude, and making the correct choices, we feel how effortless life can be. We are often told we must work hard and exert a lot of energy. But this is incorrect, because the very act of trying to force something to happen frequently negates it from happening. Why? Because force's companion is fear. Instead you need to allow events to unfold effortlessly, which happens when you connect with your intentions in the present.

Think how many times you have tried to remember someone's name. *Wait a minute. I think I have it. Gee, I almost had it.* The more we try, we still can't remember, until we give up and then it suddenly comes to us. This shows us that when we force effort we constrict energy, and when we relax we expand our energy. As our energy expands while we are relaxed, our thoughts expand simultaneously. So the intent behind our actions must be supported by our capacity to relax and to act with ease. Trying to force ourselves or others into action to reach a goal might succeed on one level, but we won't be happy with the results.

Finally, do not give power to your past. When you disconnect from the influences in your past you can then create a sustainable, successful life. The moment you surrender your power to the past, all the energy held in past memories is carried into the present. Then what happens? You discover you are remanifesting your past, literally, even viscerally. When people say they feel sick to their stomach when they think about some incident in their past, they are indeed being accurate, because every cell in their bodies holds past memories, and will hold them for the entire life of the cell. So any thought we entertain or situation we encounter that triggers a past memory, regardless of how ridiculous it might be, replays the memory all over again. Only about 5 percent of our day is spent in the present moment with clear, conscious presence. The rest of the time we are in the throes of reacting to everything, continuing to recreate our predictable patterns of behavior. Do you trust authority or challenge authority? Do you do what you are told without question or do you question everything you are told? How you answer these questions will reveal the degree you can move forward and grow.

So consciously strive to get clear about your unique, individual needs apart from other demands and reactivity, and concentrate on manifesting that positive energy. You'll be amazed as what you visualize begins to inhabit your life.

CHAPTER EIGHT

Embracing Passion

We all want more passion. Passion makes us come alive. How often have we had an experience that gives us a tingling sensation when we remember it? Try to recall all the positive and passionate feelings you've had and see how you feel. If you connect with something that's authentic for you, you'll feel it. You'll feel it in the chakras, the energy sites in your body. No matter how long ago it happened, you'll still feel it.

Every day we try to re-create sensations that gave us special feelings. Re-creating in a positive way is constructive. Re-creating by sublimating through artificial stimulants can create pleasurable sensations, but they have negative consequences. We can become addicted to sensations of all sorts, internal or external. If you spend Saturday afternoon watching football on television, you connect to the energy of what you're watching, and you feel pleasure and passion. In fact, you look forward to it all week: *I don't like my job. I'm not connected to it. Thank God the weekend is coming so I can just chill out and watch football.*

We look for ways to create connections. When you were connected to the passion in a relationship, you felt good. You were excited. You couldn't wait to be in your partner's presence because the closer you were, the more intense that intimate feeling was. And it wasn't just sexual. Intimacy is far more profound than sexuality. Intimacy vibrates at the deepest level of our being, the spiritual self. Let's take a look at what supports or blocks our ability to embrace passion.

1. Return to Your Body's Inner Wisdom

Every one of the hundred trillion cells in your body has a consciousness. If they didn't, they wouldn't know what to do. You don't tell your stomach how to digest food. You don't tell your lungs to breathe, or your eyes to blink to create tears so your eyes won't be irritated. You don't instruct your veins to carry blood to the heart at a certain rate or your arteries to carry the blood away. You don't tell your cells to take in oxygen and give off carbon dioxide. You don't tell your intestines to engage in peristalsis, that wavelike rhythmic movement that moves your food through your body and moves the dead cells, bacteria, and undigested cellulose and fibers out. How do a hundred trillion cells always work in perfect harmony and always for your betterment? They have consciousness, one that preceded life. Your mother didn't teach your heart how to beat or your brain to think. You were born with this innate knowledge, which is joined with conditioned responses and conditioned wisdom.

We're born with perfect energy and complete harmony. We enter a world that challenges us physically, sometimes with environmental obstacles like pollutants that can overstimulate and disrupt neurons. We might eat foods we're allergic to that cause yeast overgrowth, urinary problems, or ear infections. Against all of these threats, your body does something unique—it tries to protect you. It's always working on your behalf. It tries to maximize its capacity to repair the damage.

What belief system honors the body completely? What belief system says that the body and mind and spirit are intimately connected and therefore there is only one consciousness? If we understand and honor that consciousness, then we have created harmony with this life.

2. Re-Creating the Positive in Your Life

We need to recapture our passion to explore, to experience, and to allow the wonder of life that lets us wake up each day and say: *Wow! What can I experience today that is new and original?* If you don't give yourself new experiences, then all your tomorrows will be endless repeats of today, including your pain, your insecurity, and your judgments.

Every single day we have to re-create our life. To do that, we have to realize that when we wake up in the morning, we're not the same person who lay down to sleep. Our cells have changed. Our biochemistry has changed. Usually we only see change as quantum effects. We realize that we've gone from forty years old to fifty, but we didn't pay attention while it was happening. We didn't get from forty to fifty without processing changes.

The only thing we have in life is the moment we're in. We try to build lasting relationships, lasting careers, and security for our future. But the moment is all there is. When we do something meaningful with the present moment, then the next moment is probably going to be even better. If I decide to make positive choices right now, then tomorrow's choices will not be burdened by previous wrong choices. If I exercise today, my body will show it tomorrow. If I eat right today, my body will feel it tomorrow. If I think right today, my body and my brain will experience it tomorrow. If I take on the right attitude and reject what I don't want to be, I will feel it tomorrow. But it takes courage to stand up and say: *No, I don't want negative energy within me, and I have a right to reject it.* How much junk conversation and junk emotion have you taken in? You can't live off junk food. You become obese and sick. Junk relationships will sicken you too. Remember, you have the right to reject any energy that doesn't honor you spiritually, emotionally, mentally, physically, and creatively.

3. Mastering and Actualizing Your Own Energy

We have diminished the capacity to master our energy—and without mastery, we don't progress. Mastery requires the confidence to exist in the moment. It requires discipline, and the fuel that drives mastery is passion. If you are willing to combine your passion with discipline, then one day you will wake up and find you have begun to master your own energy. Your openness increases and your whole life changes for the better. But if you don't take that inner journey of focusing on the essential through discipline and self-actualization, you won't master yourself and you won't see any sustainable positive changes. We're exhausting the basic energy of our chi, which needs to be rejuvenated constantly. The chi, your central life force, can only be rejuvenated by quiet, reflective, contemplative stillness. If you're alone in nature, you're rejuvenating. If you're running around all the time, even to get your yoga and your meditation and your glass of wheatgrass juice, you end up exhausted. We need to be much more focused on how we use and direct our energies.

We wait for something to happen that will ignite our interest and inspire us to action. We want to be saved. We want to be rescued. No one is going to come and save you; you have to become highly proactive. It's your life, and you're the only one who's responsible for it. You're the only one who can self-actualize.

4. Defining Your Own Reality

How often have people told you that you can't, or shouldn't, do something because *they* wouldn't do it? Try to believe in the best you can be, in your greatest moments and in your happiest and healthiest self. Every truth starts with belief. Self-actualization by positive thought, with the right discipline, will allow the belief to manifest. I've run more than six hundred races. Before I race, I run the race in my mind so my creation becomes my reality. I focus and honor that reality. Once I was racing in the 40k National Championship Race in New Jersey with about 135 other champion athletes, the best in America in my age group. At about six miles into the race, my buddy says: "Wow! It's a hot day; this is going to be tough." Instantly I felt my energy drain out. My fatigue had started in my brain, not in my muscles.

So I said to myself. *No! This is a chance to challenge a belief It's a great day and the sun is energizing me. I want it to get hotter. The hotter it gets, the more power I'm going to have.* So I kicked in and left my buddy in the dust. People shouted out to me, "Gary, you're going too fast, you'll burn out!" But I said to myself, *No! I'm going to burn up the track. I'm not going to burn out.* I got faster and faster. When we came to a hill, I said: *Hill, you're my friend.* The hill energized me, and I raced right up it. At about the eighteenth mile, I passed the national champions in the lead and came in two minutes ahead of the second-place runner. I set a new master record.

How was this possible? Because I believed it was possible. Had I not believed it, I couldn't have created it. Whatever you believe, you can also create if you have the discipline to master it. The trouble is that we just want what we want, and we don't want to work at mastery. But simply holding a belief doesn't do us any good unless we put it to the test. Until we follow through with the reality we imagine, we won't get anywhere, and will stay stuck in our same old life.

5. We Need to Accept Ourselves Completely

Do you constantly seek success in the hope that recognition will overcome your insecurity, doubts, and fears? If so, then you will try to control everything that people think about you, through your actions and your words. You're not living an honest, authentic life. You're creating an image of yourself. If we hand over the responsibility for our happiness to someone else, then we are in a false relationship that will never work no matter how hard we try. It can be scary to think that we're so powerful that we can be complete within ourselves. We're led to believe that we're nobody unless we have somebody else or the right clothes or the right job or the right friends. But if you're fully present and you're honest, you can look for the authentic qualities in your surroundings and you can feel complete in the moment no matter what. We constantly strive for external acceptance, when the only acceptance that is important is internal. We need to love ourselves completely and unconditionally. Then what can shake you? Your spiritual and emotional roots will go so deep that in any crisis you'll just smile and say, *The universe is giving me another lesson to learn from. I'll be better, stronger, and wiser because of this.* This is all possible once you believe in the completeness of your being.

CHAPTER NINE

Change Your Life

One day you wake up and realize that you're thirty years old, or forty or fifty or sixty or seventy, and you ask yourself: *What am I doing?* Usually we only reexamine our lives at the start of these decades, almost like New Year's. At the New Year, we make our resolutions. Along about May, we realize we haven't accomplished a thing. We've started and stopped, and we're back in the same old patterns.

Now I'm going to ask you to do something different. In this chapter we're going to explore the medium in which you exist: your beliefs, your attitudes, your actions, and your emotions. I'm going to ask you to start by emptying your life, so you can understand who you are and what your life could be. Think of all the mistakes you've made. Think of all the things that have blocked you. You're going to find out what you can put in their place.

Usually, instead of emptying, what we try to do is *add*. We're almost afraid to accept that if we got quiet, faced our problems, and tried to understand their lessons, we would have to surrender some of our beliefs. Almost everything we do is based on our beliefs. What if our beliefs, or parts of them, are simply wrong? What if we changed our belief systems?

Let's begin our journey. Let's empty ourselves. Let's take everything out and see what works and what doesn't. Imagine you've taken all your socks out of your sock drawer to see which ones match and which don't. You find all these socks that don't match. Maybe you throw them away—but maybe you don't. A part of you doesn't want to throw anything away. Look in your closets. Look in your garage and attic and basement. Look at all the stuff we accumulate that serves no useful purpose.

We have a hard time surrendering things because so much of our identity is based on collecting things. We collect degrees and money and possessions and friends because that's how we create an identity. We become an extension of everything we collect. We rarely get quiet and ask ourselves, *What is the meaning of my world in relation to what I've collected? On the basis of my collection of things, am I better, or wiser, or more humane, or kinder, or more empathetic?*

What if you emptied yourself and then only put back what would serve the essential self? And how do we know what's essential when part of what we collect is our identity? Right now I'm helping a group of individuals, both men and women, who are facing a new decade of life, from thirty to seventy. I'm asking them a series of questions to help them focus on some life issues and make some changes in their lives. I'm going to do the same for you.

Step 1. Clean Out and Start Over

Think of your wardrobe. What would change if you cleaned it out and told yourself that you wanted all new clothes? I used to drive my friends to despair because every two years I would completely redo my apartment in a different style. My friends would say, "You're changing your apartment again, Gary? Why are you going through all this effort?" And I would answer, "Because I'm bored with the old decor and part of the excitement of life is creating something new." Of course it's an effort. But do you know what takes more effort? Trying to adapt to something that is boring. Another day, another dollar, and we eat the same things and go to the same places and have the same conversations. We adapt to boredom or mediocrity in our day-to-day lives.

I know many men, from forty on up, who are going through andropause. They are losing their sense of energy, enthusiasm, and passion, as well as their muscle mass. Ask such a guy, "What kind of body do you want?" The answer is usually, "How much effort is it going to take? If it's too hard, disruptive, and uncomfortable, I can't do it." So your comfort level determines your reality. You've adapted everything to a low level of discomfort. The moment a conversation becomes uncomfortable, you become defensive. The moment you could take action for change, you back off.

As each decade approaches, we focus less on what we need to do to change. We tell ourselves we're never going to be like we were, never again as young or as attractive or as accepted or as passionate. We squeeze our lives into an ever-narrower frame of existence; we hang out with people who are like us and we exclude everyone who is not. We just adapt.

Let's start over. It's a brand new day. In every aspect of your life, select something fresh and vital, from the color of your clothes, to the type of friends you choose, to what you do with those friends, to what you do with yourself, even your body.

Step 2. Examine How You Compensate for Feelings of Inadequacy

Some of the ways we compensate are by never fully relaxing, never wanting to let go, never truly being in the moment, always planning, and having to control everything. When we feel inadequate, what we're really feeling is vulnerable, and we don't want anyone to know, so we protect our vulnerabilities by disguising them. The older we get, the more layers of insulation we throw up around our deficiencies. Then we only focus on what we know will not embarrass us, what we can do with some sense of completeness. We can hide there. We can keep anyone from finding out that we're inadequate. Some people feel so vulnerable because of their inadequacies that they overeat or drink or gamble or distract themselves constantly. They even stop trying to hide it. Others are very good at hiding their deficiencies.

Everyone has mastered *something,* whether it's shining shoes or cutting hair or making clothes or broadcasting the news. But can we really grow by repeating what we do well and eliminating the very thought of what we can't, just to avoid feeling inadequate? What about the rest of life? Where is the balance? Without balance, your life will be distorted.

Step 3. Explore What's Missing from Your Life and How That Lack Affects You

To know what's missing from your life, you have to take the time to go into that conscious focus called mindful meditation. Be present in the moment and be mindful of what you would ideally like in your life. Find out for yourself: This is the kind of friend I want, the kind of body, the health, the career, the quality of time for self or others, and where I'd like to live.

Write down everything that is viscerally important to you—what comes straight from your heart chakra so you feel connected to your essential energy. Identify by name what you want and then honor it. Sometimes there's a discrepancy between our desires and our circumstances, which creates conflict: Everyone who has a desire for A but is living at C is going to feel the rub. Every day you're going to be reminded that you're not living your ideal. You can do one of two things in response. You can either 1) change so you can at least have a chance of manifesting your ideal; or 2) adapt to the pain of not living your ideal. It's going to be one or the other, and I'm hoping it will be number one. That's how we have a life. We don't allow others to tell us what we should be doing to be happy. We tell ourselves: *This is what I want. This is what I'm going to do. Here are the tools I need. Here is my plan of action.* Then don't let anything distract you.

Step 4. Ask Yourself Whether You Possess All the Resources and Openness to Change and Grow

Slow down to the speed of life. Focus with a sense of complete attention and appreciation and give yourself however much time it takes to get where you need to go; learn to accept that change cannot be rushed, nor can it be delayed. Delaying is procrastination. It is diversion. Notice how clever your mind is in distracting yourself from what you need to be doing. Look at how ingenious the excuses are. Do you say, *I don't have the tools, so I can't do it* instead of saying, *Let me get the tools I need*?

You're either going to move forward or you're going to stand still. If you stand still, watch how you react to this negative adaptation: You'll feel bitter, angry, and self-righteously indignant at the world because you're not happy. You'll blame everything on circumstances. *If only*—if only what? If only you were rich, or black, or white, or taller or shorter, or smarter? No. These are immaterial to a happy life. I know a group of people running a radio station who feel they are victims and therefore entitled to their anger. I know others who have chosen not to be victims, who have chosen to be free to create their own lives and sense of happiness and completeness. So find the attitude and the tools you need to create your own change instead of making excuses for staying stuck.

Step 5. Recognize That Distraction Diminishes the Present Moment

Eliminate distractions. The average person is now watching television for almost six hours a day. How much time do you use up in a day distracting yourself? Think of all the phone calls and chores that are meaningless. Why not just say, *I am not going to engage in anything that distracts me from what I need to balance my life.* Take all the distractions away and what are you left with? Just you. What would happen with just you? Are you afraid to find out? A lot of people can't talk about themselves because they don't know who they are. That's the result of the distraction factor.

Some people may be uncomfortable even with the idea of watching someone meditate, let alone doing it ourselves. What do they think about? How can they sit there that long? *I couldn't sit there that long. I'd get fidgety. Maybe I could sit there if I had a headset on so I could listen to music; then I could do it.* But that's not meditation. Meditation involves being present and saying: *No more distractions.* We've created all our distractions because they're such useful tools to keep us from making transitions.

Step 6. Confront the Fears That Come with Change

Change cannot come without risk. Think of how many times you wanted to do something different but first you had to get the approval of others. Why do we think we have to get approval? What is it we think someone will say? They might say, *Yes, go ahead and take that class. Take that vacation.* But what if we wanted to do something unexpected? What if you were a successful lawyer and you said, *I'd like to go out to New Mexico and spend time with nature.* To do what? *Nothing.* You're a three-hundred-dollars-an-hour lawyer! *I know, but I want some hours to do nothing, to charge nothing, just to commune with nature.* This step will be so radical that you're going to think you need help from others.

First ask yourself which you are more afraid of: the change itself or the oppositions and confrontations that arise when you're seeking another's approval. If you want to be healthy, why should there be an argument about it? If you're sick and seeking an alternative therapy, why should your doctor say: *No, you can't have a second opinion or a third opinion or an alternative opinion.* Why should the doctor be concerned? Why shouldn't you search out different opinions so you can look at your options and grow? Usually we play it safe and only ask those authority figures who assure us that we can make a decision on their say-so. Think of how many times people vote or eat or dress or work on the basis of what others say is best for them.

When it comes to change, the risks have to be faced. We need to see a situation for what it is. Only then are we ready for true healthy change. If we keep looking and distorting and repackaging and reframing and refocusing because the change is not acceptable, then all we're doing is playing the game of manipulating illusions. When we feel uncomfortable about making a change, we avoid it or put a pretty face on it. Hopefully, one day we will wake up and say: *Why am I doing this?*

Step 7. Learn the Lessons of Your Crises

We need to see ourselves in a different way. The way we do that is to learn the lessons of our crises. Every crisis carries its lesson. Let me give you an example. I know a woman approaching forty (let's call her Cynthia) who invited a troubled friend (let's call him Joe) to stay with her. Cynthia is an activist in the peace movement. The situation with Joe is stressful, and she frequently blows up: "This guy gives me no privacy and is very jealous. He wants to know every place I go. But I can't ask him to leave—where would he go? What would he do?" I suggested she ask Joe what he intended to do with his life (which had nothing to do with her life). Then I asked her what she intended to do with her own life. She wasn't having a relationship with Joe. He was the man who came to dinner and never left. She said, "I know, but—."

Then I started to realize that Cynthia was getting much of her sense of self from taking people home so she could rescue them. She needed to be needed. Why? Because she believed that her value as a human being lay in saving people. But was Joe growing and changing? If you have someone staying with you for a year and you're taking him to yoga and meditation and nature outings and he's no different, then it's time to reassess. He hadn't changed. He had just gotten a year of free room and board and hanging-out time. Joe needs to get out and support himself. Cynthia is caught between two worlds: anger at her loss of freedom and autonomy and the need to show that she's caring and nurturing. What are the results for her? Refortification of an old belief system. And Joe? He hasn't been truly helped, and he hasn't changed.

When we learn the lessons contained in our crises, then we can grow. Any lesson you don't learn you will repeat over and over again. The universe is good about giving us many lessons. Sometimes divorce, bankruptcy, separation, or loss is the lesson we've been given. We get angry when these things happen, and we don't look for the how and the why. We just think: *Get me out of here!* But along with the pain and suffering, we have something to learn. When we can pass the test because we've learned from a lesson, we probably will not have to experience the same pain again.

Step 8. Appreciate Your Life Now: Don't Wait for Loss

I know people who start anticipating their losses as they approach certain decades. *I'm hitting fifty and I can never think of myself as young again. I'm hitting forty, and the gray hair is coming in.* I just talked with a woman of forty-nine. She said that her libido had been nonexistent for the last year. I asked her why. She said: *Because I'm forty-nine, Gary. What guy gets up in the morning and thinks wow, I really want an aging out-of-shape forty-nine-year-old? No. They want young women. They want what I was when I was twenty-five and sexy and fun. I'm accepting it.*

Accepting what? Accepting that because you're forty-nine you should no longer have a libido? You should no longer be passionate? You should no longer allow that chi to flow? You should forget everything you can still do? She said yes. I told her that by cutting off these energies she was going to manifest a limited life. She said she was not alone. I said, no, you're not, but what if I showed you a woman of forty-nine or fifty-nine or sixty-nine or seventy-nine still actively enjoying her sexuality? Still seeking ways to explore it and expand it and enjoy it? She said they were just being immature. Her belief system told her that at a certain decade she had to adapt to a preconceived social notion, "act her age," and close down her sexuality.

When we do this, we're honoring everyone else's beliefs about ourselves. How positive is it to think that when you hit fifty you're going to be less than you were at forty or forty-five? That's not a healthy mindset. So enjoy what you have every day because if you took away the calendar and no one knew how old you were, then age would just be a number. What if you lived your life as if age were only an insignificant number? Then you wouldn't adapt to preconceived notions of what you should or shouldn't be doing at a certain age.

Where I grew up, by the time you were thirty you were already supposed to have a family and be well along in the job that you would have until you retired. Not too much new was supposed to happen. Maybe by thirty-five you could upgrade a bit because you could afford more. You were looked on as a mature part of society. It was expected that you would join the Kiwanis or the Jaycees. You'd go through the usual transitions. At forty you'd start to slow down and take it easy. You'd be a coach, but not a player. You'd expect to have the potbelly and the high blood pressure and the diabetes and the heart disease. By fifty you would be looking at retirement places. You'd feel satisfaction because you'd gone to the Grand Canyon five times. Where was your life in all that? Oh, we're solid as a rock and about as exciting.

We have a whole nation of senior citizens acting like senior citizens: We'll go putt golf now, but not too strenuously. We'll exercise just a little because we're senior citizens now. No libido for us. Society minimizes a whole culture, saying: *You're no longer relevant.* You don't have to accept the rules of this game. Break the rules. Just be a living human being who does not care what age you are.

Step 9. Consider What You Have in Abundance

Think of the things we all have in abundance. We have an abundance of people we can share positive energy with. We have an abundance of nature to enjoy, an abundance of love to give and receive from our companions. We have dogs, cats, birds, and fish for pets. We have an abundance of energy to focus on what we can bring into our lives—hobbies, skills, new tools. We have the wonderment of how many things we don't know. Even the knowledge of all the PhDs at a major university is like one grain of sand at the bottom of the ocean floor.

If all this abundance of things to learn and to experience is there for us, why do we act as if we're paupers—emotionally, intellectually, and physically? It is possible for us to live in the abundance of everything that we can embrace. Think on that the next time you start feeling insufficient and incomplete. It's like a person saying: *I'm starving.* You say: Here's a buffet of three thousand foods that are all healthy. *But I'm starving.* Well, dig in. *But I'm starving.* Pick it up. Try it. *I can't.* Why? *My belief system won't let me.* It's our belief system. Our belief system is our reality. We'd rather starve emotionally and spiritually than connect with the abundance of energy around us.

Step 10. How Can I Go from Here to There?

How can I go from where I'm at to where I need to be? By realizing that you already have everything you need to take a step. If you're approaching or are sixty and you want to feel sixty, then you'll feel old. You'll feel less. You'll feel loss. You'll feel that a whole lot of life is behind you, only to be remembered by scrapbooks and occasional flashes of inspiration. Or you can say: *I don't care how old I am and I don't care about the circumstances I've accepted. Today I am focusing my energy in this moment on what I want to experience and I will seek out the tools. For every tool I seek out I will surrender a tool that no longer works.* Surrendering the tools that no longer work releases the energy that goes along with them.

When you sacrifice to find meaning, the meaning will have purpose. The fear of sacrificing what you now have means that all you will have is what you've accumulated up to this point. Ask yourself whether the sum total of all you've accumulated represents the blissful peace of mind that you are seeking. Look at all you've accumulated and ask yourself what you would surrender to change the energy. When you surrender what no longer works for you, you automatically empty out that energy field to bring new energy in, whether it's people or ideas. That becomes your new energy. That becomes the new medium.

Don't allow your truth to be distorted by the bias of another. My truth works for me. Throughout my life I've never felt that I fit in anywhere. So instead of trying to remold myself to fit into the narrow confines of society, I've chosen instead to expand my consciousness to wherever it would take me. Although there were risks, sacrifices, and pain, I know what is possible because my freedom took me to the top of the mountain and I saw the future. People's fear so often keeps them in the valley, and all they see is what's right in front of them. Think of the difference. I know you want a fully realized life, and this is what you can say to yourself:

I am more than my beliefs. I am present for my own creation. Every day I choose to re-create myself over again in the eyes of myself and not the world. I do not get my view of life through the eyes of others. I can see myself for who I am and what I want to be. It's through my own eyes—my spiritual eyes—that I see my journey ahead. It's society that sees my journey from behind.

I'm either going to look ahead or look behind; I'm going to look with my eyes or theirs. Their eyes are going to be aligned and unified, and their strength will become my weakness because their strength allows me no independence and no autonomy. If I choose to look at life as a medium to which I can surrender by emptying out the negative and filling it with the new and the positive, then I'm taking a step that they're not going to take. They will hit forty, fifty, sixty, and seventy and be angry or depressed or look in a mirror and consider woefully what is no longer present. I will look in the mirror and say: See the potential of what still is.

CHAPTER TEN

Choose Your Lesson in Life or the Universe Will Choose It for You

D o we choose our lessons or does the universe choose them for us? When we are in school, learning is very straightforward and easy; there are no tricks to that kind of education. But what happens when we are tested either by the choices we make or by the situations the universe puts in our path? And what happens when we pass or fail these tests?

Teachers in school systems across the nation impart information that they believe is important for a student to learn. Students are then responsible for learning and assimilating what they have been taught. Today teachers will sometimes even tell students what will be on an exam, and the students pass according their different levels of proficiency. But does this really prepare anyone for anything essential in life? In most cases it doesn't.

Every day we are given challenges and we need to know how to pass them. Unfortunately, the majority of us do not know how. Even worse, we are not diligently seeking the lessons that enable us to grow. There is a long story I will share, a true story, which exemplifies very well the principles in this chapter. The story's content and situation may not reflect your life exactly, but it is very instructional about how tests are faced in life.

There are two people in a relationship who I know very well. Over the years both of them have shared their stories and journeys with me. I have known the woman, who I will name Joyce, for about three years. The man, who I will name Tony, I have known for much longer. Joyce is very creative. She loves the arts and music and believes she can become a talented singer. Her heroine is Andrew Lloyd Weber's former wife, Sarah Brighton, a very gifted classical performer. Joyce plays the piano and some guitar. She is loyal to her work at menial jobs but is bored and feels that whatever she accomplishes is not good enough.

Joyce was in a relationship that was stagnant, a dead end, but she held on steadfastly. There was no joy or pleasure in the relationship, only constant quarreling and neglect. Because Joyce grew up in a family that believed if you make a mistake you must stick by it, she remained obligated to the relationship. When I asked her if she was happy, she replied that she was miserable.

Joyce put all the gifts she felt she possessed on hold for the sake of the relationship. In other words, she gained a relationship but lost her life. A quality relationship is one where there is no judgment, no attempt by partners to change or limit each other, and where the individuals are accommodating in order to be themselves and to be free to grow.

Joyce would tell me, "Gary, I would love nothing more than to be a free soul, to live my life as I really want. I need private time, and I don't want to be questioned about where I am going, what I am doing, who I met or called. I don't want jealousy from a possessive man who is so insecure that he feels threatened if he is not involved in everything in my life." Joyce was assuming that the man she was with was the only man she could be with. If she felt otherwise at times, guilt and shame arose, which only made her try harder.

Think about how often you have heard people say, "try harder." Or they say, "Not everything is perfect. We don't have the best relationship but at least we have stuck it out," as if that will win them the door prize. So many relationships today subsist on suffering. The partners no longer feel they have anything in common. Communication dies because they feel they know what their partner will say before she or he speaks. Nothing is new in their lives and there is only the repetition of eating the same meals and acting out the same routines. This is not a quality relationship. It is a hardship that people take pride in because they have stuck it out. If you ask these people to run in a marathon, they will respond that they could never endure it. Yet they are enduring far worse by running a marathon in their relationship every day of their lives, except they are blistering their souls instead of their feet.

Joyce had a very dominating and dismissive father while growing up. He showed no unconditional love and found it necessary to demean his daughter in order to make her feel unworthy, a dynamic she felt in her current relationship too. So when Joyce had the chance to make a break she leaped at the opportunity.

Having freed herself from her obligations, Joyce soon wound up in a relationship with Tony. Tony is about as different from Joyce as you can imagine. He is a James Dean type of guy: easygoing, nonaggressive, accommodating, a super-cool rebel. He takes risks to experience things most people otherwise fear. He doesn't blindly accept barriers and limitations. In short, Tony simply likes people. And now Joyce was beginning to have new and exciting experiences through him.

Joyce, Tony, and I arranged to get together. I asked Joyce how she had been doing. "Oh, I can't believe it," she said, "I'm doing all these things I have never done before."

"Well, how do you feel about it?"

"At first I didn't quite understand it," she replied, "but then I just let it happen and I started to enjoy myself."

One day Joyce and Tony showed up at a race I attended. Joyce won her race, which was very impressive because she had become very serious about exercising only recently, and for the first time in her life she had won something. Tony was so proud of her when she had the gold metal placed around her neck. Then she ran another race and won again. Afterwards I asked Joyce how she felt.

"Gary, I'm so excited I can't tell you. I really did this on my own and I feel great. I am motivated to train now. I just wanted to do something that would break down some barriers." Then she started listing all the barriers she had broken down.

"That's terrific," I said. "Now, would you have broken all those barriers if you were just on your own?"

"I'm not sure."

So I continued, "Joyce, be careful not to mistake experiences, no matter how good or bad they feel, for your own growth if those experiences are motivated, inspired, or impassioned by someone else. You could be using someone else's energy as your own."

When I spoke with Tony I told him the same thing. I also said, "Tony, you have to understand. If you are a dynamic energy and very active in pubic, you might have a dozen or more people living off your energy and you won't be aware of it. While you might think you're motivating and changing people, and might think they are transforming because they're in your presence, that is only your ego speaking."

Dynamic men and women will always draw nondynamic people toward them. It is as if these dynamic individuals are a light and wherever they go there is an illumination of body, mind, and spirit.

We feel terrific in the presence of such people. We are like a cold child coming into a warm room when we are around illuminated individuals. The key question is: Can we understand that these people are giving us a lesson? We can only learn what a lesson has to offer once we have taken ownership of it. In other words, we have to create the lesson for ourselves over and over again. It must become a regular part of our lives until the day arrives when we are no longer connected to the people who originally inspired or motivated us. If we have taken ownership of the lesson, we become inspiring and motivating ourselves.

Be careful that you don't mistake mimicry for self-actualization. There are so many people who mimic the beliefs, words, and deeds of those who inspire them, but the moment the person leaves the room the light in their life dims, and they revert back to their old self. There is nothing to sustain us when we revert back to the time before the lesson was given.

There was a period of about three months when Joyce, Tony, and I were in frequent communication. During this time I had an opportunity to clearly observe the dynamics being dramatized both between them and individually. Here was Joyce desperately seeking to discover herself through another person. For his part, Tony gave Joyce the freedom and opportunity to explore herself. Without criticism or judgment he provided a vehicle of unconditional acceptance for her to experience life on her own. Although Joyce managed to do this, at the same time she was unable to learn from the lessons. She had mistaken the experiences for the lessons. The lesson is about how we *grow* from the experiences. Do you understand the difference? Never confuse an experience for a lesson. That is the reason we all have countless experiences but continue repeating the same mistakes.

One day Tony seemed concerned about something. I asked what the problem was. He said, "How do I know that Joyce is really happy? I just have this strange feeling that something isn't right." I asked if there had been an argument. "No, but it's almost too good." I asked him why he couldn't just accept a positive relationship. A few days went by, and then he called me with an interesting story.

Two nights earlier Joyce and Tony had gone on a trip together. Joyce was feeling spacey, apparently because she hadn't eaten, which was putting her on edge, and they started getting fractious with each other. Tony said, "Joyce, I would rather be alone than be with you when you're in a bad mood." As he was walking away Tony added, "I really don't want this energy." But what Joyce chose to hear was, "I don't want *you* in my life ever again."

Isn't it interesting what people will hear? This is what the conditioned self heard because that is the self that always seeks the exit doors in life. When insecure people take a step forward with a new experience, the conditioned self starts planning an exit strategy. There can never be a full unconditional commitment to anything as long as the conditioned self is always looking for an exit strategy.

Insecure people frequently look at experiences from a vantage point of weakness and fear. Regardless of what face they wear— giddy, happy, excited, merry, open—part of them doesn't believe a situation is really secure. Because they don't believe a relationship is real, the mind seeks a way to escape. For example, how many times in your life have you experienced that people or friends you work with disappear when you confront a crisis in your life? Immediately they are gone. One small episode and they vanish. When we use our intuition we can observe how and why this is happening.

The following morning Tony apologized to Joyce and reconfirmed his commitment, love, and respect toward her. Later he told me, "Gary, it is as if one evening I'm holding this warm beautiful rose and the next morning I'm holding an ice cube." Joyce had severed the energy between them immediately.

The following day Joyce had already moved out, not only physically but also emotionally. When I asked her what her feelings were, she said, "I don't want to be around anyone who is going to be hot and cold toward me." So I said, "From what I understand it has always been hot between you. What you experienced was taken out of context. We are given tests in life and the way we respond will determine whether or not we're growing. The issues you confront will determine the quality of your character, your integrity, decency, and ethics, and your determination as a human being. If you fail this innocent test, how will you respond when the test is more serious?

"The good news," I continued, "is that you haven't been with Tony long enough to have wasted both of your lives. So where are you going to go now?"

"Well, you know, I'm going to be around other people."

"Oh, so now you are going to take this guy who cared about you and throw him aside as if there were a better relationship just waiting for you around the corner? Who else will give you unconditional freedom to be who you are?"

Whenever life offers us an opportunity, we should seek the lesson in it. Some of us do everything to avoid and deny lessons by remaining firmly entrenched in our old belief systems and behavior. We delude ourselves into believing that we already know and do the important things so we don't need to learn anything new. But where does this get us? It keeps us right where we have always been.

Only by changing something fundamental in our lives can we evolve beyond our present level. All of the energy that keeps us in a static condition is adaptive energy. It is not transcendent energy. When we begin to move beyond our current level of energy to seek lessons that challenge us, we begin to perceive the truth of who is real and honest and who is not, and the reasons why. Think of how many times we simply assume that someone in a business partnership or relationship is honest and will not betray us. We believe them because we have conditioned faith when they say they are honest. Later they turn out to be untrustworthy or they betray us.

Everything important I have done in my life is the result of my seeking and finding the lessons to be learned. Sometimes I failed the tests I confronted. Yet when I fail I pause long enough to remove the ego so I can relearn from the test even if it is unwanted or painful. The healthy approach to difficult tests is to say, *Okay, I really do not want to have to learn this lesson again. I want to just learn it once, and no matter how many times I am tested I know I can pass.*

Very often the challenges and tests I am given try the very core of who I am. You do not hear me attack someone or defend myself on the radio or Internet because I was attacked—although I receive some e-mails assailing me. When you are happy and no longer insecure, there is no further need to waste your energy talking about your story and defending yourself. When you are not preoccupied with your story you can live life. All of life then becomes your story and every day you open a new book to write a new tale. There are always new adventures and excitement because each day is a new story that has nothing to do with yesterday. Every day there is growth because there is no longer anything holding you back.

CHAPTER ELEVEN

Rebalance Your Life

Health is a balance of our emotional, physical, and spiritual conditions. At the cellular level, life is a constant struggle for balance. Even when you ingest what is harmful, your cells will always defend you. They never stop and say, *Why should we defend this guy? He doesn't care about us. He's abusing us.* All of the hundred trillion cells in our body are operating on our behalf. Each of them has a separate consciousness that works in unity with the others. We overeat, and what do the cells do? They could put all that extra weight onto the nose, but they don't. In a miracle of balance, we put on a little weight here and a little weight there. Why? To keep our center of gravity in balance so we won't fall over. Because the body is seeking to create balance, people rarely become disproportionately fat. When we don't take in enough calcium, the body tells the kidneys not to secrete too much calcium, and it also adjusts the sodium levels. Every second of our life our body is adjusting our biochemistry based on what we've done to it, often quite harmful things. When we smoke a cigarette or drink alcohol, the body rushes in a whole army of immune modulators and other defenders in an attempt to protect and rebalance us. That's how wonderfully intelligent the human body is.

Balance is one of the keys to life. We need to look at every part of our lives to see which parts are out of balance. These will be our problem areas. When you spend more than you make, you're financially out of balance. In a relationship, if you take more than you give, you're emotionally out of balance. When you give more than you receive, you know it; you know you're with someone selfish and your needs are not being considered.

Have you ever been nodding off to sleep while you're sitting up, and suddenly you jerk yourself awake? You were losing your balance, and your body was trying to get it back. If the outside air is smoggy, we close the windows. If the water is unclean, we filter it or drink bottled water. If our body is dirty, we wash it. Everything we do is an attempt to compensate for some lack of balance. But so much imbalance exists that we begin to take it for granted.

The body and the mind never take imbalance for granted; they're always working to keep us healthy. The body and the mind want you to have emotional, physical, and spiritual balance so that the best you can be emerges. We can also fool ourselves that moderation is balance; that's what most people think of as balance. But think of being okay with a moderate amount of sarcasm, or negativity, or racism, or sexism. Do we ever say, *You can be racist one day a week, you can lie to me occasionally, and sometimes you can betray me?*

What if someone says to you, *I intend to cheat you and lie to you and betray you and talk badly about you and steal from you and give you a disease, but not all the time.* You're not going to answer, *Oh, thank God. I thought you'd mistreat me all the time.* No. You would turn from such a person because you would see the problems, instantly and intuitively. The relationship could only get worse, because once something is out of balance, it always gets worse. Generally we only pay attention after the crash. We almost have to break down to break through.

Many people refuse to clean up their act until they're forced to. Suddenly they're in front of a judge: *I'm sorry I got drunk and I'm sorry I stole. It won't happen again.* Why did it have to happen at all? Because even on a mental level, we don't honor who we are. Until we honor the real self, we're going to think in an imbalanced way. How can we change this? How can we create an ideal balance in our lives so everything flows?

When you're working with effort, it's almost always because you're out of balance. When you're in balance, everything flows. Your mind flows. Your body flows. Your spirit flows. You don't have to think about being nice or wonder who you're going to be nice to. Everybody gets the benefit of your niceness and your love and respect. When you have to wonder whether you should be helpful or kind, you're still in conflict.

So where do we begin this journey? We begin with an exploration of some issues. You provide the responses. If every single one of you had a different response, you could all still be right.

1. Positive Defiance Creates the Freedom to Be Yourself

What would change if you were defiant? James Dean represented defiance, and so did Marlon Brando. Certain people have always stood out because they refused to toe the line. They were defiant. It's one thing to be defiant simply to draw attention to yourself. It's another thing to be defiant because you are unwilling to compromise a principle. Our society keeps telling us to compromise on essential principles. What if you chose not to? What if you chose to be the defiant one? What would you stop doing? Choose something you can be defiant about and then draw a line and say: *No more compromises.*

Every year on New Year's Day I take a careful look at the people in my life and I ask myself, *Do I deserve to be in their life? Do they deserve to be in mine? What are we sharing?* How often has a friendship or relationship that was positive at the beginning gotten progressively worse after all the damage and dysfunction in a person are revealed? The next thing you know, you're just another caregiver for someone who's using the relationship to unburden themselves on you. If I'm defiant, I will say, *You can bring me your ideas and your energy and your love. Do not bring me your garbage and dump it on my psyche.* Because of guilt, shame, insecurity, and uncertainty, we're tied into these rituals of trying to save people who don't want to save themselves. In part, we're trying to redeem our own life by taking on the suffering of others.

Why not be around the millions of people who are happy and healthy and positive? You have to choose positivity. You have to project it. You're only going to get what you project. When I was told I was no longer appreciated or wanted on a certain noncommercial radio station, I immediately projected out to the universe that I wanted to continue sharing and to connect with people who could understand and share with me and not act against me. Calls came in from everywhere: *Gary, let's do this, and this, and this.* Every day I'm going places and I'm talking with positive people because suddenly I'm no longer associated with a negative, toxic energy.

You can't connect to two things simultaneously. You can't be happy and sad. You can't be positive and negative. You can't be honest and dishonest. So look at your life and see what you have connected with up to this point, because that is part of the problem. You can learn how to separate yourself from what you no longer want so you can be free and open to associate with something that you truly want. Forget the past. People keep digging through their past like emotional archeologists, looking for the remnants of a broken relationship and a dysfunction they can understand and define.

But what if we simply accepted that we're living from today

forward? I can't do anything about my past, but I can do something about right now, and so can you. What do I want today? I'm going to be defiant, constructively and positively. I will stand up for a principle. I will not allow negative people in my life. I will not abuse my body, mind, or spirit.

2. Finding the Courage to Say Yes or No

When have you said *yes* when you really meant *no*? When have you said *no* when you should have said *yes*? Think of all the times you didn't feel confident or complete enough to take hold of an opportunity in the moment it occurred, so you turned it down. Sometimes you said yes because you were expected to, or someone convinced you to. Think of all the choices you made because you were told there was no other choice, or you didn't deserve another. Some people will go out and marry the first or second person they meet, as if they'll never have another chance.

One day you wake up and find that you're forty or forty-five, or fifty or fifty-five, and you think: *I'm glad I've gotten what I have and now maybe I should pay attention to self-actualization.* That's when you begin to think carefully about what you're going to say yes or no to. Ask yourself: *Will saying yes or saying no bring back balance?* With balance comes positive energy. You surrender the negative energy of imbalance. You surrender one to bring in the other. No matter what's happened in the past, if you bring in the positive and surrender the negative, you can start over today. Today you can say yes to what creates balance and no to what does not. *Do you want to take away my time, be negative and dishonest?* I say no. *Do you want to share love and kindness?* I say yes.

How often have people said nothing out of fear of the consequences? How many of the 748,000 doctors in our country had the courage to speak up for the few who were stepping into the wilderness to blaze a path in alternative medicine? Our trailblazers were immediately attacked by the Food and Drug Administration, the state attorneys general, and medical boards. The innovators weren't prepared for a fight; they were peacemakers, not warmakers, and they were helpless. They had the interest of the patient at heart, and pioneered with great character and courage. Their colleagues, who hid behind their insecurities, will one day have to come to grips with the consequences of their silence.

When you know you have to speak up to maintain your balance emotionally, do it. Silence in the face of apartheid, racism, sexism, or any form of human rights violation is wrong. I don't have to tell you that. But we have to find the courage to say no. Right now, as a nation, we can't find that courage. We're allowing misguided people operating from the wrong values to make choices for us when we should have the courage to make our own choices.

3. Change Nourishes Your Vital Force

We like to think that we always stay the same. When we buy clothes, we don't think that next year they'll be out of style or we won't fit into them. But life changes every second of every day, like a wonderful stream that's flowing forward. Why do we dig in our heels and say no to change? Because it's uncomfortable. *Get me the gated community. Get me the consistency. I don't want change.* Like it or not, everything is changing constantly, at every level. Wouldn't it be better if we simply allowed ourselves to change and controlled the change, rather than end up a victim of what we did not choose to control?

Recently I was on a television program and the host said to me, *Gary, do you really think you can get most Americans to give up their bad habits so they can be healthy?* I said, *It's not my job. It's their job to give up bad habits. It's my job to let them know about*

the positive outcomes that are possible. We only go through one of
two doors in life. If you open one door, all you're going to get is
older. You'll go through multiple pauses: menopause, andropause,
brain pause, thyroid pause, prostate pause. The biochemistry changes,
and the body begins to slow down, imperceptibly at first. Then you'll
become more and more prone to disease. You don't have to be clair-
voyant to see the outcome. Sickness. Disability. Diminishment. Because of medical advances, some of us can reasonably expect to live
into our nineties. But we're not going to be in vital health. We'll be
lonely and dilapidated. What are people going to do with all that
time if they don't have a zest for life? How many Jerry Springers
and Oprahs and Pizza Hut commercials can you watch before you
want to scream? When you are existing passively, living the exact
same life day after day, you get bored and depleted.

If you open the other door, your life will be completely different. You'll be in a flow, one that you're controlling. You're controlling what goes into your body. You're nourishing the skin to keep
it young, nourishing the muscle system to keep it strong, nourishing the brain to keep it thinking and creating and challenging. You're
always looking for an engaging adventure. You're not waiting for
life to reward you or rescue you. You're actively engaged because
you know that balance comes by going forward and making your
choices based on the outcome that you want. You don't have diminishment and disease. Instead you have vitality, renewal, and change.

How often have you felt you didn't have a choice? You were
stuck in a job or a relationship and you had to carry your burdens
for years. Let's say you're now in your forties or fifties and your
family is grown and gone. For better or worse, they're out there.
You've done what you're going to do with your career. You want
something new. Maybe you want something new sexually. You're
thinking about it for the first time in years. You want different kinds

of friendships, more engaging friendships, with people who can challenge you. You want to see the world. You want to visit new countries. You want to open yourself up to other cultures and other people. You want to learn a language. You want to move. You want to give away all the stuff you've collected. Now you can do it, because there are no more excuses. If you *don't* change, your life will no longer work for you.

Now let's say you're twenty to thirty. You're in transition. You're figuring out what you can do. You're putting all your energy into your work and into proving yourself. It's the proving decade. Between thirty to forty, you're trying to figure out what you want to do now that you've proved yourself. Usually you're going through the anxiety of trying to accumulate enough stuff to make yourself feel good or prove to others that you made the right choices. *See? I didn't waste my life. Look at what I have—the car and the house and the bank account. That's me.*

Then, in your forties, you look at all this stuff and say, *What the hell is all this about? Why am I here? Who am I?* By fifty, you're thinking: *Am I three-quarters through my life? Am I all washed up?* In our society, Hollywood producers are not looking for us.

We're a society in which people are separated off by decades and discouraged from making changes. *Come through this portal. Don't go back. No more disco dancing. Don't act young anymore. You can't dress that way. Look at your hair. You can't get away with that.* You start realizing that society wants to dictate how you dress and how you move and how you act. Society wants to artificially separate people, races, religions, and cultures. It's no wonder people are confused when they go from one decade to the next; now they don't even fit where they did before.

When I first came to New York, I worked briefly at a Fortune 500 company. It was there that I saw I could never work for a big corporation. I'd rather be unemployed or self-employed and take a chance—I just didn't fit in. I actually don't fit in anywhere. I don't fit in corporate America, or in government, or in industry. I don't fit in movements because I don't like the egos or the lack of balance and the mindset of most people who run movements—not that the movements don't have legitimacy. I can believe in a movement; I have just never believed in most of the leaders.

At this Fortune 500 company, an older woman sat at the desk across from me. She had been there for forty-five years. Some of the other long-time employees gave her a party when she retired, and then she was gone. It was a sad goodbye. About a month later she came back to say hello. No one wanted to know her any more. It was heart-wrenching; I was watching her trying to make conversation with her old friends, and was seeing them thinking, *I've got to get back to work. You're no longer a part of us.* That woman had given her entire adult life to a company that no longer gave her a moment's consideration. She was part of the past and not the future. And she was lonely—she may not have developed any outside interests. When we get disconnected like this, apathy is the next stop. Seeking out change, even in little ways, can keep us from becoming too rigid in our life.

Don't go along with the foolish notion that you've made your bed and you have to lie in it. I renew everything I do on a monthly basis. If I've made inappropriate choices and decisions, I can disengage from them. Embrace and seek out change, and you will discover a renewed vigor for life.

4. The Rewards of Risk

What are you willing to risk? When I spoke out and was thrown off a radio station I had been on for twenty-six and a half years, was it worth it? You bet it was. By taking that risk, I disconnected from people who did not appreciate the energy I was giving. Now I can connect with people who respect my energy. So much of what I do is risky. Here's how it works: No risks, no rewards. Little risk, few rewards. Big risks, big rewards. You've been playing it safe. You don't do anything without guarantees and assurances. I don't do anything *with* guarantees or assurances, and I don't have a fear of failure. In my world, there is no failure, there is only a lesson. If I make a mistake I can learn the lesson it offers and then realize, *Because of this mistake, I am stronger and wiser and more humbled and humane.* Therefore the mistake is a strength and not a weakness. Don't be afraid to take risks, because otherwise nothing will change.

5. Unnecessary Demands Will Drain Us

We all know how often we've felt we had to honor a certain demand. It's another ball we're juggling. One day we've got so many balls up in the air that our whole life consists of juggling responsibilities. And we're afraid to let go. What would happen if you let all those balls drop? You could pick up the responsibilities that are ethical and important and let the rest be.

Learn to say no to all the demands on you and your time. Take back your time. People will say you're selfish. In reality, you're selfless because you're honoring the eternal self. When you have more time because you've given up unnecessary responsibilities, you'll have more freedom. You won't have the excuse not to self-actualize.

I recently counseled a woman from Long Island who has a serious autoimmune condition. She had been to four different holistic doctors. When I asked her about her life, she said, *What does my life have to do with my condition?* I replied, *Let's talk about it, and maybe we'll find out.* She told me she had three sons living at home who were seventeen, nineteen, and twenty-two. She was doing all their cooking, cleaning, and laundry, and she was giving them money.

I asked her why they couldn't do all that for themselves. They would show they cared about her if they said, *Mom, you don't have to clean for me. You should have your own life.* They were selfish— they were allowing their mother to do what they were capable of doing for themselves. But her mind was so fixed on the concept of caregiving that she couldn't even conceive of taking back her time. Because she never has the time to focus on her own needs, she is always stressed out, and the stress creates an elevated cortisol that adversely affects her immune system. So she's walking around with a broken-down immune system looking for a nutrient. I told her that the nutrient she needed was self-love.

When I'm running on the beach, nature is energizing me. When I'm meditating, I'm being energized. My pets energize me, as do good music and the gourmet meal I've just created. Say no to unnecessary demands so you will have the time for energizing experiences.

6. The Dreams of Youth Are Possible Now

Remember the dreams and fantasies, hopes and desires you had when you were younger? Revisit them now and ask yourself how you can turn them into reality. It's important to have dreams and fantasies and inspirations; the mind can take hold of an inspiration and project it out to the universe. Then you can connect. You can't hold your thoughts in and expect a connection.

Back then you didn't have the resources to fulfill your dreams. You didn't have the knowledge, or the character development, or the ability to take risks. Now you do. Now you have nothing to lose. You can make your own desires important.

Have you outgrown your life? I'll bet your life could be far more dynamic and complex than the narrow confines you've stuffed it into because of a limited belief system. You've let someone else tell you that all your values and beliefs and inspirations and qualities must fit neatly in here. But your thoughts are out there, far beyond the confines of your life. So, like a snake shedding its skin, surrender the old self and emerge with the power to be who you really are. Live as big as your life is. Stop trying to fit a size twelve foot into a size six shoe. It's painful. It's the pain of constant conformity to society and its ways, which you don't even like. You've become frustrated, angry, and finally depressed. So spring back. Have a life that's as big as your ideas. Revisit those wonderful dreams you had earlier in your life and make them happen.

7. If Our Problems Are Learned, They Can Be Unlearned

I believe that many of our problems are learned. We learned to eat the hot dogs, the hamburgers, and the pizzas. We learned to gamble and drink or take drugs. All our learned activities and beliefs have consequences. What if you examined everything you've learned and asked yourself, *What do I want to unlearn because it no longer supports my sense of self, my balance, and the ethics I want for myself today?* How do you unlearn something?

Look at the consequences of your beliefs and ask yourself whether you want them. If you don't, then surrender that belief. It will free you up to learn something that is more essential and authentic in the moment you're in. Then you can go forward with your life. You can't go forward with old learned habits that no longer suit you. You can't drag this stuff along behind you into the future. You have to go forward unburdened.

8. Learning the Right Lessons Takes Courage

How can you discover the right lessons for you? By figuring out what it is you need to learn, not being afraid of it, and actively seeking it out. If I want to learn the lesson of health, I have to study health and then I have to participate. I have to self-actualize. If I want to learn about courage, then I have to act courageously, including saying no when I would otherwise have said yes. That takes courage.

Think of the power of believing in what's possible, believing in yourself, believing you can achieve your desires. You can overcome illness. You can heal relationships. You can find the energy you want to connect with. Believe in yourself, not the past. Believe in now and in the future. Put the energy there and stay strong. You're telling your cells, *Cells, I believe in you.* The cells, all hundred trillion, are answering you, *Thank you. You caught up to us.* Now you're believing in the totality of life, projecting out the energy that you want and allowing in the energy you want. The negative energy can pass right through you.

At the end of the day, we'll wake up and make a choice. Our choice will create either balance or imbalance, harmony or disharmony, disease or wellness, happiness or sadness, constructive or destructive thoughts. It's all in your power. You can make it happen.

CHAPTER TWELVE

Enhancing Self-Esteem

Our success, or what our society defines as success, is more often than not determined by how far we climb the social ladder to achieve prestige and wealth without having to expose our vulnerabilities, insecurities, and fears. In our highly competitive culture, we frequently find someone seeking a way to take advantage of the very thing we are trying to achieve or resolve. Our right hand asks people to be open and genuine. We appreciate it when people expose themselves honestly, but if we are not in a balanced spiritual place our dysfunctional alter ego will manifest itself, and our left hand will seek a way to take advantage of people when they are honest. As a result, people become fearful and distrustful of others. They may close down and eventually become less likely to be open about their inner thoughts. Even as we seek balance in our lives, we often still habitually engage our world and ourselves in an imbalanced manner, and in the process our self-esteem suffers.

Let's explore the question of self-esteem more deeply. Gautama Buddha told his audience to listen attentively to his suggestions, weigh them carefully, and afterwards adopt only what worked, discarding what didn't. Authentic individuals past and present who have offered advice to others have given that same caveat. The suggestions I will outline are only based on my own life's experiences; you need to decide which ones resonate with you and which do not. Hopefully the information I share here will trigger some insight and illumination that can help you put a spotlight on your problems so you can see them more clearly.

When we have difficulty being open and honest with others, we compensate by stepping back from a person in order to assess the circumstances and what the person is thinking. What we may be doing is looking for a way to be accepted. Acceptance to win someone else's favor then becomes more important than our frank honesty. In most cases, our calculated interpretations of circumstances and people are misguided, hence our conclusions are erroneous. We discover ourselves being misunderstood and this leads to frustration, self-doubt, and a lowering of our self-esteem.

Ask yourself this question: What real value am I to others, such as family members and friends, if I have not done the things that are truly meaningful to my own existence? If I can't be responsible and caring toward myself, how can I be a pillar of kindness to loved ones? Instead of discovering our true meaning inside ourselves, we turn outside to society and hierarchical authorities to conform with conventional social expectations. Everyone we associate with, every institution we affiliate ourselves with, has different expectations from us. But what do we expect from ourselves?

We are told that there is a love for us somewhere out in the world and when we find it we will feel better about ourselves. We believe that if we can find it, hopefully by just bumping into it, our self-esteem will flourish and we will then have mastery over our lives and feel fulfilled. But we shouldn't be looking outside of ourselves for that which is already naturally inside us. The journey to discovering self-esteem is a completely internal process. Mixing up a sojourn that is real and internal with an external hunt for the pot of gold at the end of a rainbow will never bring the positive results we want for our self-esteem.

For example, we look at models and actors, people in power and authority, and we think how nice it would be to have their lives. But do we ever seriously consider at what level we want to emulate them? Are we really aware of the suffering that celebrities and people in authority go through? They do suffer, but their internal suffering is hidden unless it gets played out publicly. The idyllic illusion of celebrities' lives becomes the delusion we have about our own existence, and all the while we continue to dance around trying to figure out who we really are. Each of us needs to pause long enough to take an honest look at our authentic selves. Next, we need to deconstruct each and every part of ourselves that is unreal in order to uncover who we truly are, removing the corrosion hiding a beautiful statue. Perhaps untruths we identify with are real to our employer or maybe to our friends, but they are ultimately unreal and false to us. Until we are authentic to ourselves we will continue to live an empty existence.

First and foremost, we need to experience and understand the very foundation upon which everything within our being resides. How do we do that? During the quiet moments of each day, select one question and investigate deeply how it applies to yourself and the life you live.

Do you possess all of the resources and openness of character to make a firm decision to change and grow?

Begin by making an honest and detailed inventory of everything you are: every personal quality, moral character, social value, habit, and conditioning. Your list should also include every attribute that defines an authentic self for you. Then reflect on each item in your list attentively and note whether you possess it or not. For example, courage is an important attribute for living an authentic life. Without courage, how can you accomplish anything truly worthwhile and noble? How can you stand up for higher values in the face of adversity without courage? Without courage, you are unable to break away from the past, with all of its conditionings and unhealthy patterns, in order to accept and embrace who you really are. There comes a time when you need to face what you have become as a result of being inauthentic in your choices and actions and say, *That's not me anymore. It used to be me but today I am someone else.* Everything that limits your self-esteem needs to be abandoned, and courage enables you to do that. You no longer identify with the past because the past is dead. It ceases to exist. Moreover, once you have accepted your authentic self, you need to constantly call upon your courage to sustain your authenticity in every life situation and personal encounter you meet.

If we want to make fundamental changes in our lives, it is imperative to seek the truth in everything. Only then will we find the clarity and inner resources to make the critical life changes. Ask yourself whether you have the determination and motivation to seek truth regardless of how deep you must dig. Do you have the courage and fortitude to stand up as a freethinking human being and challenge the artificial social environment and the people who wish to curtail your growth and imprison you in their false belief systems? It takes impeccable honesty to acknowledge that something that appears to be real is inherently false. These are the essential qualities—determination, courage, fortitude, and honesty—to create authentic self-esteem. Such self-esteem will vibrate differently than your usual manner of living and dealing with situations because you will be observing all that is artificial as a spectator instead of being immersed in it as an actor or actress. When you learn to become an aware observer, you will discover truth and meaning in everything.

There are many reasons why we fail to master energy. Among the most common reasons are a lack of self-confidence, lack of discipline and control over our bodies and minds, and our lack of self-esteem. Once we are able to accept ourselves completely, including all our gifts and all our foibles, then we discover self-esteem. There is no better way to enhance self-esteem and harness its benefits for living an authentic life than by accepting the self, because then we are not centered in our ego and trying to legitimize the ego's desires. Whenever we try to validate ourselves to someone else we are falling into a trap of losing our connection with our true self. You could be absorbing the energy of the other person you are trying to convince of your worth. This is a cause for arguments, conflicts, and fighting, and more often than not, counterproductive. Our self-esteem should be based on that which is authentic for living a productive and healthy lifestyle and not on that which is only superficial.

The majority of our emotions find their origins in our past. We drag along so much baggage into every new day as if it will help us survive, but when we discover it is unable to serve our immediate needs, we enter a macabre course of suffering, believing that suffering will redeem us and restore our self-esteem. However, there is little redemption through suffering. If something happens contrary to expectations and personal desires, we may withdraw into imbalanced emotional responses. It might be anger, anxiety, or depression. Where did we learn this? From our past. That is why it is so necessary to understand your past and find the courage to separate yourself from the energy of the past's influences. Unless you remove yourself from the past, it will continue to manifest in your behavior, emotions, and mind. Much of your mind chatter will be little more than a continuum of inappropriate reactions out of sync with your true self.

Is the life you are living too small and limited?

I firmly believe that the vast majority of people in Western societies live a life too small and far below their full potential as creative and self-actualizing human beings. One reason for living a small life is because other people exert their unconscious fear upon us as soon as we stand apart from them and take the initiative to expand our horizons beyond what they believe is in our best interests. When we try to justify all of our decisions from a small, compartmentalized box handed to us from our childhood, and later from education and society, we cut ourselves off from feeling and experiencing life's deeper meaning. During our growing years, we were instructed that every answer to our questions was found inside the prevailing paradigms and their spokespersons. Eventually we realize that we are not being listened to clearly and those answers are not really helpful.

It is so important to come to the clear realization that most of our lives are influenced by the energy from our past and the energy of other people. While we have all had our positive, blissful moments—a bonding of love, communing with gorgeous scenery, or moments of childhood wonderment—we have also had our many moments of pain and suffering. When our life and thinking are too small, when we are too sensitive to the powerful influences of others, our defense mechanisms are weakened and we simply absorb the energy around us. Remember that making fundamental changes in your life can be instantaneous because truth is available at every given moment, free from past and present negative influences.

Building Self-Esteem through Focus and Mastery

Create a list of every thing—minor, moderate, and major—that you want to change in your life and behavior, select one thing, and remain absolutely focused upon it, giving it your full attention. Simply keep yourself present in the moment with that one thing you want to change. Each day, throughout the day, keep your attention on it until you have mastered it. Eventually your attention on that item will drop of its own accord when you have become what you focused on. At that moment, your mastery will vibrate within you. Then move on to another selection on your list and repeat the same process. The important thing to remember is to only focus on one item at a time. If you are trying to do more, you are multitasking, which diverts your attention from mastering either. I am constantly working on many projects but I never lose my sense that I am my most important project. Every day I make sure that I have what I need to maintain my balance. I come first in my life because if I am not at my optimal state of physical, spiritual, and mental health I am not of maximum benefit to others. Because I come first, I will not permit myself to make any excuses that will jeopardize my health. As a result, I remain in a balanced state of mind with passion, commitment, and determination to accomplish whatever I am undertaking, and my self-esteem remains high because I am vibrating with positive energy.

Suppose I did not take care of myself and continued to live and work at my current pace. For example, what if I become so absorbed in making a film that in my rush to finish it I didn't bother to eat well? And then there are the people I want to counsel and books to write. I would be working from eight in the morning until four the following morning without giving myself proper nourishment, exercise, and rest. Within six months to a year, my immune system would start to collapse. I would be out of shape, toxic, and stressed. For whose benefit can I then be helpful? The very thing that I have dedicated myself to do—honoring my life by helping other people honor theirs—I would be unable to do. My fear of not being able to live in a way that is meaningful for other people would manifest. By taking time to be attentive to everything important in my life and being honest about whatever presents itself before me, I can sustain my balance and self-esteem.

Consider the vast number of people who believe firmly that they will earn respect in the workplace by working a dozen or more hours daily. Then there are millions of people who believe that if they can take care of everyone else's needs they will prove themselves as responsible caregivers and win appreciation from others. These are erroneous ways to build self-esteem. The proper way is to focus on you. When you treat yourself with tender loving care, what you need to do for others will become effortless because there will be no conflict or contradiction in your decision about what should be done. Separating the illusion from the reality of your life is going to save you a lot of time and disappointment.

Think of something that you have exerted an enormous amount of effort on only to discover that you gained less than you expected. It might have been a relationship or a job that you ended up devoting yourself to until one day you realized it wasn't right for you. The reason you may feel you were left with so little for your efforts is because you were building the relationship or project on the conditioned self and not the real, authentic self. The good news is that when you become aware of it, you can begin to change the situation, whereas before you didn't know how to because you didn't have the proper tools. By focusing on one issue at a time and sticking with it until it is accomplished, we can develop the tools and skills of awareness.

Identify all the things in a single day that you have done and that are a reflection of yourself.

Everything we do in our life is a reflection of ourselves. Give yourself some time to think about all the things you do during the course of a given day as though each is a full expression of yourself. Next, ask yourself whether you like what you see. If I am mirroring myself and my actions, I want to see how I have been displaying my authenticity. During the day have I been kind, thoughtful, loving, and compassionate? Have I been caring and nurturing? If I do not witness any of these attributes at any time then something urgently needs to be changed.

There is a great danger in changing only your perception about yourself without changing your actual self. So many people across the world only change the perception of themselves. This is like mastering the art of illusion. In some shamanic cultures, particularly in South America, it is called shape shifting. But in our case, there is no true mastery of reality involved but only manipulating one illusory shape for another. The danger in only changing our perception and not working on changing ourselves is because it is a form of lying. Those who master this art are prone to deceit and betrayal, even when they know it is wrong. They refuse to acknowledge the mirror of themselves as a thief, liar, and betrayer. All they manage to do is alter their perceptions of themselves so they can accept the illusions they create in the mirror.

The task before you is to see yourself for who you truly are. Be willing to go through the discomfort and even the pain to take a hard look at yourself in the mirror and say, "yes, I have identified with these negative qualities and I don't want to continue doing things the same way." Believe it or not, you can do this with acceptance rather than making it an exercise in lowering your self-esteem. The attitude with which we approach our assessment makes all the difference.

It is far healthier for you to be aware of yourself with all your weaknesses and negative energies, because only then can you start to make real, progressive change. It takes a great deal of commitment and discipline to create an authentic self. By doing so you discover authentic self-esteem. Because true self-esteem does not require applause, adulation, approval, or ego stroking, you will discover a passion to seek only for what is most authentic in life. In that journey you will remain in the moment and fully live your life.

CHAPTER THIRTEEN

Perfect Harmony

I believe every single problem we face, whether in a relationship, a job, or our physical and psychological health, can be reduced to one simple question: Are we living in harmony with ourselves and our world or not? This applies not only to each of us as distinct individuals, but to entire groups, societies, and even nations.

The ego has a brilliant capacity to rationalize and create excuses for not doing what we know we should. We are the total accumulation of everything we choose in life, and in most cases we are the embodiment of excuses keeping us addicted to the foods we eat, a life full of multitasking, lack of exercising the brain and body, and unhealthy habits. Therefore, we need to step outside of our conditioning, become present to the moment we are in, and with deep conviction ask ourselves whether our lifestyles and habits are making us healthier or sicker, happier or more depressed. By doing this, we challenge the ego and put it into a dangerous situation because the authentic self we are all born with inherently exists without confusion. The authentic self will only make right choices for us.

It is comforting to believe we are progressing. But what is important in life? Progress or something else? What is important is happiness, health, joy, and loving relationships. Yet we are unhappy, unhealthy, and our relationships lack meaningful quality. Three hundred more schemes for improving our lives will not suffice. Another film like *The Secret* will not change anything essential. These are gimmicks keeping us distracted from ourselves because the majority of them are instructing us to do something outside of ourselves: connect with someone or something else such as new guru, the next marketing entrepreneur of personal motivation ploys, or the next pharmaceutical cure. None of this helps to fundamentally improve the quality of our lives. We make wrong choices and act inappropriately, and this hinders progress. By their nature, bad choices arise because of our defense mechanisms, which is why the pattern of inappropriate choices is repeated over and over again. The only proper remedy is to make right choices, act accordingly, and then honor those actions. In order to do this, we need to surrender everything that causes wrong actions and then become increasingly consistent in doing what is correct. When we make a mistake, we must be honest with ourselves and acknowledge our erroneous decision for what it is.

Everyone who lives in denial of their poor choices eventually becomes angry when the consequences of their actions catch up with them. They are angry at others or themselves, and this leads to self-loathing. They will blame others for not warning or stopping them. There is nothing constructive to be gained from blaming others and loathing oneself. Instead it benefits us to understand the reasons for our bad choices and how we exchanged good energy for bad energy.

Everything in life is an exchange. Every thought, every word, and every deed is an exchange of one energy for another. Therefore it is essential to understand how energy is exchanged when bad energy is substituted for good energy. Only when you surrender the energy that leads to conflict can positive energy enter in and help you grow and mature spiritually so you no longer feel limited, imprisoned. This is the way to master the art of *not-learning*.

I believe our culture is largely uninterested in real learning, because if we were actually learning we would eat better, think more clearly, treat each other with kindness, and not dull ourselves with numbing entertainment like *American Idol* and *The Bachelor*. We have no essential need for commercialized garbage. There is no aesthetic or cultural value in violent films and programs. So why do we watch such drivel? What purpose does it serve? These programs are only distractions barring us from fully engaging in the wonders of life and reaping life's rewards. Compulsive attention on relationships is also a distraction. I live on the Upper West Side of Manhattan where there are many restaurants. Whenever I go into one, 90 percent of the people I overhear are discussing problems in their relationships or why they don't have one. The story line is always the same: why don't I feel good about myself because of another person? Only on very rare occasion do I hear someone musing about the possibility they might be living an inappropriate life and making wrong choices. And never do I hear someone stating they need to surrender something negative in their thoughts and lifestyle to achieve something better and more authentic.

When you observe people who really want to make a positive change, you will see that they put a halt to their mental and emotional games and commit to learning more about themselves. Such people say, *From this day forward, the only choices I will make in my life are the ones I want to be a part of me in the future.* When you dedicate yourself to this kind of thinking, you no longer compromise. When you cease compromising you begin to rebalance yourself. Restoring balance in your life is simultaneous with a refusal to make compromises in favor of the negative, and focus on sustaining the positive.

One of the dangers we face today is everyone's need to be right, competing with each other to prove their superiority. The need to be right in whatever you are doing derives from the need to maintain control over another person or the situation you find yourself in. The need to control always leads to conflict, tipping the scales into a state of imbalance. A true sense of being right comes from a natural evolution of decisions and actions that avoid conflict. When you place yourself in the right situation there is no disorder, disharmony, and disease. So be wary of associating yourself with anyone who has a need to be right.

The need to control is a sign of a deep unhappiness. Why aren't we happier? With all the money people are earning, with all the technological gadgets and commercialism, with all the advanced telecommunications to connect us with others, why is there still such dissatisfaction? Happiness is a natural state of being. It is not something outside that you need to hunt for or strive to earn. As long as we can simply be in the present moment, we have an opportunity to feel happy and blissful. I don't need any "thing" to make me happy. If I lost everything I own, I would lose nothing that deprives me of inherent happiness. My life is more essential than a house or the clothes I wear. My life is more significant than the money I make. So don't approach life and the pursuit of happiness from the fear of loss, because if you fear losing something then what you fear is what you will actually manifest.

When you start your day without fear in your heart and your mind then everything is possible. There is no need to control or manipulate anyone or anything. The need to play games with the lives of others disappears of its own accord. To simply be is a marvelous state where something unique and special happens. There is a sense of ease and peace, a satisfied comfort with yourself, and a radiating sensation of love. When you are in that state you are able to manifest the life you were always meant to live.

My old ranch in Texas was a beat-up place. Nobody else wanted it, but I felt completely at peace there. For that particular time in my life it felt like the right place to be. The universe, when you open yourself up to it, tells you where you ought to be. So I accepted this disaster of a ranch and fixed it up. A year later I opened it up and as many as one hundred people would attend any given retreat. We held sweat lodges with the Choctaw Indians, offered saltwater scrubs, and all the participants had a wonderful time. At night, I would look up into the starry sky and feel a oneness with the universe and everything around me. During those moments there was no need to prove anything. I only had to be present for my own life and live it authentically and honorably. That is harmony. And the amazing thing is that when you are living in harmony, you attract others who are also living a balanced, harmonious life. Like seeks out like, not through any concerted intention but simply as a natural and effortless unfolding of life's events. When you discover there are hundreds, even thousands of people, sharing the same positive rhythm, the world is no longer a cold place. You are not alone. You love and feel loved because your energy expands and intensifies by connecting with others whose energies are synchronous with your own.

Conversely, imagine going to a concert hall and sitting with a hundred other people, all playing an instrument sounding their respective lives, no one in harmony with anyone else, creating a cacophony. Each of us is a combination of millions of energies, including not only each vibrating cell in our bodies but also the energies of our family members, neighbors, colleagues, pets, and home. You have to harmonize with each of these energies as well as with the processes of your body, including aging and illnesses. You have to harmonize with the causes you espouse, your religious beliefs, and your social and political values. There are so many things you have to adapt to in order to say, *I am a good person*. Indeed, in one area of your life you might be a spectacular human being but that alone does not translate to mean that your life is in harmony. It only means that there is one level where your energy is not conflicted. But what about the other parts of your life? Even if the greatest pianist in the world were to play on a completely out of tune Steinway, his playing would irritate us.

Everything in life is interconnected, therefore you need to work on every area of your life. Replacing one worn washer of an engine that is otherwise in need of a complete overhaul will not bring the engine to maximal performance. Everything important to you can be traced back to something you have given allegiance to, including the beliefs instilled in you as a child, the ideas imprinted on you by teachers and bosses, and the illusory carrots held out to you by popular entertainment, the media, and politicians. Locate the origins of your allegiances. What are the beliefs and values they represent, and why have you connected with them? Are they constructive or destructive? The answers will not come easily. Succeeding in this exercise requires patience, so allow yourself time. We are usually so occupied with the angst of our being that we keep ourselves unknowingly distracted 24/7. We are either on the phone, mindlessly watching TV, or frantically completing a project or chore. Distractions console our fear of being simply present with ourselves. When you stop everything—all distractions, all noise, all meaningless contact with others—there is only you. Once you are fully present and feel happy and at peace with yourself, then everything else you have aligned with is seen for what it is: illusions to distract you from being present with your true self.

You can't take a sliver of this and a chunk of that and call your-self whole and balanced. This is a warped way of bringing us into harmony and balance. It is incomplete and will never prove successful. Many people rush off to yoga retreats, spending their days twisted in postures, but their minds are somewhere else. Shoppers in health-food stores buy bags of wholesome foods, but the rest of their lives can still be unhealthy and imbalanced. Reading Deepak Chopra's books doesn't make you automatically spiritual; taking Andrew Weil's advice and getting a colonic won't make you completely healthy.

Not only do we need to act in ways that harmonize our lives, we also need to hold inspired thoughts. Hundreds of thousands of great minds throughout history have left a legacy of inspired thoughts for our benefit. For a full day, take an additional step in harmonizing your life by reflecting only on harmonizing thoughts. You can find examples from Spinoza, Maimonides, Gandhi, or even your grandparents, parents, or siblings who left you with wise words at some time in your life. Or you can give it a go and create your own inspired thoughts. You will find life flowering in more wondrous hues as you delight in holding inspiring thoughts in your mind and imparting them to others.

Do not expect the answers to your disease and dis-ease to come from today's institutions, government agencies, and media. Ultimately you are the only person who can make the important choice of staying positive and focused on that which will help you. Think of the story of the Chinese official sent to meet the young Dalai Lama during Mao Tse-tung's reign. When the official tried to convert the Dalai Lama to the liberating values of Maoist Communism, the young lama replied, "You cannot liberate me. I can only liberate myself." You need that kind of conviction to bring harmony into your life.

Finding true harmony requires developing a sense of independence. You can begin by deciding to build a sustainable life for yourself. How many of us are unable to sustain our relationships, our health, our expenses, and our lifestyles? The precariousness of our lives on a razor's edge creates anxiety. If something is not sustainable, do not support it. If you are engaged in an unsustainable situation that is creating stress and confusion, let it go. First work on what is immediately within your means to sustain. You can make the transition from disharmony to harmony overnight. The way to master accomplishments is to master one area at a time, and with each accomplishment you increase your positive energy, strength, and fortitude to tackle the next area. So begin with the area in your life you can engage and connect with most easily. With each accomplishment you are going to feel like a new person is being born.

Next, reflect upon how each day you struggle with the conflicts and crises of yesterday. Give up yesterday's crisis; in fact, surrender yesterday altogether. If today you meet someone you had a conflict with yesterday, change the energy of your relationship in that new meeting. Simply smile and say, "hello, how are you doing today?" Today is a new day; yesterday is gone, just a memory. Don't allow the memories of yesterday to conjure yesterday's feelings and turmoil. When you act in this manner, you will discover an alchemy that transforms not only yourself but the people you have difficulties with.

Every morning wash your mind clean. Surrender your biases, your prejudices, your anger. Every thought is the beginning of a wave of energy. Focus on what you need and how you will chose to think about it. Align your feelings and thoughts so that you are in balance. Then project those positive thoughts out into the universe and be prepared for the returning energies that you can align yourself with. This allows for the harmonizing of more life forces to accomplish what you alone may not have been able to do. Remember, harmony is possible only when you believe in the completeness of yourself.

CHAPTER FOURTEEN

Prescription for Your Soul

There have been many discussions of self-empowerment by good people who inspire and motivate us, such as Wayne Dyer, Deepak Chopra, and Tony Robbins. I suggest that in addition to the benefits derived from those sources you become your own coach. This practical self-inquiring approach works well for the people I counsel. See if it works for you.

What is normal? Socrates said, "The unexamined life is not worth living." You are the only one who can really examine your life. Part of a wholesome regimen for your soul is to take inventory of your beliefs to examine the actions and limitations that your beliefs produce. Let's begin by asking a few questions. Go to neutral. Take a deep breath, and be 100 percent honest with yourself. Be candid. Are you a leader or a follower, or a balance of the two? Balance is key. Most people conform throughout their lives, believing they approach the mirage of perfection by blindly following the general consensus or norm. So ask yourself the question, "What is normal?"

Where I came from in West Virginia, normal was family sharing meals together every day. You had a chance to exchange ideas and argue things out, and there was the comfort of fitting in with caring, loving people. Our fellowship at the table was an example of the supportive family structure we had in West Virginia, which was good, but the way we ate was not so good. It was considered normal to eat until you were full because someone in China might starve if you left any food on your plate, so I would say, "Well, send them what I'm not eating." I was thin and wiry, didn't have a big appetite, wouldn't eat meat, and I was fanatical about germs. If anyone sneezed at the table, I'd just refuse to eat. My brothers, sneezing intentionally in my direction, often enjoyed my portion of dinner. Everyone was expected to make fun of the whole idea of germs. When you did get sick it meant some kind of bug was in the air that everyone was going to catch. We never thought that what we did, the choices we made, could contribute to how our bodies processed disease. Again, that was normal. Nobody really paid attention to hygiene, especially where I grew up.

I also noticed that protesting during the Vietnam War wasn't considered normal behavior where I grew up. In fact, speaking out against authority was not normal behavior. Challenging belief systems was not normal either. We were taught good things, of course, such as basic morality, the importance of decency, honoring your word, being trustworthy, not stealing, and loyalty. Those things were important, and they still are, but in hindsight, there were just too many things we did that were considered normal that were not right.

Ask yourself how many damaging things you do simply because you're told it's normal to do them. Which of these behaviors, if examined honestly and carefully, would you find inappropriate or unnatural?

Here's a cautionary true story: Eve went to her doctor and he prescribed synthetic hormone replacement therapy. Eve quickly phoned her friend, Claire, to ask if she was taking synthetic hormones. When Claire said she wasn't, Eve (a true follower of her peers) threw the prescription away. On her next visit, Eve's doctor asked if she was taking the hormones. She said, "No." He continued to goad her to take them for a year, but she did not. Then on a recent visit, Eve asked, "Doctor, how come you've stopped trying to force me to take the hormones?" The doctor smiled and said, "Oh, they're not in style now." What he did not tell her is that it had been proven that synthetic HRT (hormone replacement therapy) can kill. What would have happened if Eve's friend had been taking HRT? Are you one of the women who still believes that synthetic hormone replacement therapy is required for your health and beauty?

Conversely, consider how many life-enhancing things you do not do because you think it is abnormal to do them. For example, think of how many people in America over the age of forty do not exercise regularly, and how many over age eighty don't exercise at all because they imagine they are too old. Yet it is true that the older you are the more you need regular exercise to stay well. The disease process is going to be more systemic if you don't exercise. We can absolutely trace the rise of diabetes, obesity, dementia, Alzheimer's, and Parkinson's disease to people who don't exercise and don't eat healthful foods.

Am I encouraging you to tear up your doctor's prescriptions? No. Am I telling you to trust your friend's medical advice? No. I recommend that you empower yourself by finding reliable up-to-date sources for your health information to supplement (not replace) your physician's guidance. You needn't follow authority blindly, nor peers blindly, nor just guess. Do your own research. Read. Ask questions. Get the facts and balance what you know with what you intuitively feel is the best course of action for you. That is empowerment.*

---

* Through my Web site, www.garynull.com, you can access my live Internet and radio programs for dependable health updates, search an extensive audio (and article) archive, and read the latest health news, all free as a public service.

Is the need to fit in worth the cost of following the majority blindly? If you're eating the normal diet, expecting the normal life span, and exhibiting normal behavior, you're not going to feel very comfortable challenging what is considered to be normal, are you? Suppose everyone else says we should be at war somewhere, but you wonder, "Well, really, should we be at war?" If everyone else tells you it's the right thing to do, do you think, "Who am I to speak out against it?" Would you find the courage to protest if your child's life were at risk?

There are times when you will know that it is appropriate to rebel, as exemplified in this compelling true story. Joe and Phil grew up together in small town America. They were best friends. When the war came, they were in the same battalion overseas. One day they were bombed, and Joe was able to rush to safety. He realized immediately that Phil was missing and might be trapped. Joe asked Captain March for permission to return to the site under fire to rescue Phil. "Are you crazy?" Captain March replied. "You'll be killed. I forbid you to go back there!" Joe turned on his heels and raced toward the devastation, disobeying his commanding officer. Soon Captain March saw Joe hobbling toward him carrying Phil. "I told you!" Captain March shouted, "I knew he must be dead!" Joe replied softly, "He was alive when I reached him. His last words, smiling, were 'I knew you'd come back, Joe.'"

Almost every benefit in life appears to be based on fitting in by following orders without ever questioning them, conforming to the prevailing standard operating procedure no matter how arbitrary or even deadly it might be. Hence, millions of people throughout the world devote their lives to perfecting the appearance of being just like everybody else. Do we ever really grow up, or do we just continue to copy others as children do? Ask yourself if the need to fit in is worth the cost of obeying the general consensus blindly. Think it through before you go for a full-body CT scan that delivers an estimated dose of radiation to your lungs and stomach that is "equal to one hundred chest X-rays or one hundred mammograms," according to Dr. David Brenner, Professor of Radiation Oncology and Public Health at Columbia University.

What would happen to you if you had no safety net? Think of all the people in America who would have had to declare bankruptcy if they hadn't had someone who cared enough to lend them money. How many more people would be destitute? Fortunately, in many cases, people are there to aid you both financially as well as emotionally, with encouraging advice.

Unfortunately, this assistance may make people think twice before challenging the status quo. There is a risk in being dependent on anyone because if you express independent ideas you may alienate them. If, for example, you believe, based on reliable medical data, that vaccinations may harm your child, you may need courage to take this position vis-à-vis your family and friends. The best safety net is made up of people who care about you enough to respect your rights, including your right to think for yourself, and who will not abandon you for being honest with them. It is safest, of course, not to ever need to rely on family or friends as financial safety nets, but such sensible autonomy might be considered abnormal.

How in the world are we ever going to improve anything in life unless we can clearly distinguish what is normal (an arbitrary cultural construct) from what is right? Quite frankly, I don't care about what's normal. I care what is right, and there is often a big difference between the two. Remember, for a long time it was normal to be a racist. It was normal to have slaves. It was normal to believe that women should not have the right to vote because their brains were thought to be smaller than men's. And long after African Americans finally got the right to vote, it was normal to continue to prevent Native Americans from voting. *Why should we trust the Indians with anything?* was normal thinking—prejudiced, but considered normal. Were there exceptions? Yes, but the majority of people define what is considered to be normal. The fact that a consensus agrees upon something does not mean that it is right.

Carefully consider the complete spectrum of what you believe is normal, from your diet to what you watch on television, to how much time you spend on the telephone, to your politics, to your religious beliefs, to the kinds of friendships you have, to how you view what you should be allowed to do at different stages of your life. Deconstruct your assumptions, ascertain artificial limitations you have placed on yourself and on the abilities and options that you think you have.

Recently there was an article in the *New York Times* about a man in his late forties frequently partying with women in their twenties. He was considered particularly unusual because he was going to dance parties. Well, so what? Dancing is part of the joy of life. Do you believe that it is normal for people over forty to associate only with people their own age, never with younger or older folks? Should they also go out only with people of their own economic status, at their own educational level? What if we started dealing only with people who look like us? Caucasians with Caucasians. Hispanics with Hispanics. Uneducated with uneducated. Under this rubric, if Gandhi were alive today, with whom could he socialize? Do you know any skinny, humble, poor old men with a loincloth? Start thinking about how absurd it is that we should be so limited because we want to be normal. We're afraid of not fitting in somewhere. Why are we so fearful of being unique?

Our insatiable need for acceptance is debilitating to our true self. If anything will hold you back, it's needing the comfort, support, and constant validation of others. It means you don't feel authentic on your own; that you may be so self-conscious that, like a teenager, you may be unable to just enjoy life without worrying what everyone else thinks of you. Do you know what happens when you allow yourself to enjoy life? You become secure. You do not feel threatened. You're just happy and you're sharing your joy. Some will connect with your joy, some won't, and some will be intimidated by it. The "normal people" may find your vitality downright disturbing, especially if they don't have any.

It's paradoxical that we fear our own individuality, which is the very thing that makes us worth remembering. That wonderful crazy thing you did that was so incredible is what you and your friends all still laugh over, right? You don't get together and say, "Hey, let's relive those monotonous conversations that bored us, and the movie we walked out on." You don't remember what was most bland. You recall the high points. You can become remarkable if you show up for your life. It's important to focus on how you can have exceptional experiences—because it's the best meal you've ever had that you remember, not the Weetabix. Now the problem for most of us is that the older we get, the less these high points occur. They seem to happen when we have enough enthusiasm to fully experience life and create something pleasing to recall. Wake up in the morning and say, "Hey, I'm feeling good, and the rest of my day is only going to get better!"

You can create a peak moment if you know how to do it. First, learn how to recognize what is not stellar. Living every day as if it doesn't matter is not stellar. Living every day as if it's okay to just get through the day with your pain, suffering, depression, or anxiety, most of which we could change to make way for better days, is sub-stellar. Children have exhilarating experiences all the time because they are free, honest, and innocent enough to enjoy the moment they are in, until they become corrupted by following our dreary example. So let's put "Show up for your own life!" high up on our to-do list.

Think how often you've thought of going to a play or to the opera or of doing something spontaneous, but no. *No, I'm too tired. What if I fall asleep? I don't know the outcome. There's no guarantee I'll like it. There might be a stampede during intermission.* Uncertainty or fear turns us into robots cruising through life on stagnant autopilot routines. Start asking what you can do to revive yourself. It's when you make your life vital that your natural passion for life returns. Turn that flame up, the foundation on which almost all of our energy rests, and as it starts to revive you begin to attract other people. Just the intention to do something unique in and of itself attracts other energies to you.

It's the energy you project that counts. It's not about your looks. It's not about your weight. It's not about your nationality or race. It's not even about your age. That's immaterial. Do you think Picasso was ever considered boring for all of his eccentricities, from his rageful violent moments to his sublime artistic moments? Was he out of balance? Frequently, but at least he lived an engaged life. There's no excuse to take a backseat to your own life. Why retreat?

Charles Dickens's most autobiographical novel, *David Copperfield*, begins, "Whether I shall turn out to be the hero of my own life, or whether that station will be held by anybody else, these pages must show." What do the pages of your own life show? Are you the hero of your own life, or are you phoning it in and constantly disconnected? Regular people create exceptional lives. We're not born great. You create your own great life, and to create yourself you have to get out of the way of all the clutter that prevents you from being you.

Actualize your intentions by choosing worthy goals, and using only worthy means. Now here's a path toward success: achieve worthy goals by using only worthy means. If you wish to achieve something that honors who you are, you must visualize it clearly. The intense focus on what you want, seeing the picture of it, painting it in, is like taking a canvas and showing yourself your ideal house. You cannot obtain what you cannot envision. Imagine this is your ideal relationship. Visualize the ideal body you would like, and then create it. You cannot hope for something to change if you don't know what it is you want. What good does it do to be free from something if you don't know what you want to be free for? You know you don't want to suffer, but if you're not sure what you want instead, you'll be stuck in no-man's-land. So always look to your future and see exactly what you do want. Visualize what you need. Master that visualization, and when you've mastered it, project that energy outward. As that energy unfolds it becomes a wonderful tidal wave that sweeps up the energies of other people, and the wave returns to you enhanced.

It's amazing what can happen when you send positive energy out into the world, but if you are afraid or defensive, if you're uncertain or anxious, you only send out fearful energy. It's like having guards with guns surrounding you: you may feel protected, but you will also be unapproachable. Vulnerability opens the door to the exchange of energy; fear closes that door. Love and hope open to potential.

Think of your goals and of the many ways in which you could

achieve them. Take no shortcuts. Do not use any means that are deceptive. Don't use people in any way in which they may feel betrayed or exploited. Do not meet your needs at the expense of others. You could wish for wealth and engage in unethical activities to get rich, and just be selfish with your wealth. Without a cooperative approach you will fall into using unworthy means.

What is missing from your life? Ask yourself this important question. Focus on what you don't have that you really need. How many times do we see only what we have, like our wealth or our work or our friends? It's fine to be thankful for those things, but that is not what is at issue. Always focus on what you're missing that is essential to your well-being. That is where you must direct your mind in order to progress.

Draw power from the inspiring, motivating examples that surround you. About fifteen years ago, a man named Terry Fox, who had lost one of his legs to cancer, walked clear across Canada, showing that regular people can be heroic even through great adversity. We love it when someone who seems to be at a disadvantage comes from behind and surprises us. But it also reminds us that we sell ourselves short constantly, settling for less than our full potential.

Movies can also inspire us, like *Seabiscuit,* about the horse that was broken and damaged but came back to beat War Admiral, considered to be the greatest racehorse of his time. Seabiscuit inspired our whole nation in the midst of the Depression to have confidence, hope, and even optimism. The Pimlico stands were packed to the rafters with waves of thunderous cheers as Seabiscuit, who was so down and out and thought to have no chance, came galloping into championship history to become a beloved American hero, winning against all odds and setting a new track record. A film may inspire you and, at least temporarily, help alleviate your troubles. What inspires you can motivate you to see things differently or take more risks. Seek out what inspires you. All you have to do is look around you each day; inspiration is everywhere. Go to the bookstore and pick up a biography of someone you admire. It's important to remember that everyone, no matter how great, has weathered difficult times and persevered.

Do you actualize your intentions? If you do, you'll achieve even more than you ever expected. If you see your mistakes as opportunities for learning, you'll realize your goals that much faster. Every time you achieve something you didn't even expect, you're going to wonder, *My goodness, I did this. How did I do this?* And then you'll accomplish still more. Like compound interest, the momentum of success building on itself can sometimes be staggering.

Last year in Boston when I was at the Indoor National Master's Championship, I noticed a woman training who had a perfect physique and long, beautiful blonde hair. She looked about thirty-five years old. Later that day, the same woman raced, and she set an American record. She was seventy-two years old. Seventy-two! Her face and body were naturally flawless, and she looked happy. She ran and walked with a great sense of ease. She wasn't holding the problems of the world in her; she just surrendered tension. When you surrender the problems of the world, you're free. And when you're free, you move freely. Your energy is free; it flows, it inspires.

This woman first had to choose an intention, and then she had to be aware enough to ask, *All right, I have an intention. Now how can I go from this intention, which is just a thought, to self-actualization? What tools do I need? Do I need discipline? Do I need determination? Do I need to overcome fear?* Seek out the tools that you need and begin to implement them. Never look at a mistake as a setback, but as a learning opportunity. Depersonalize. Disconnect from being harsh or critical or in any way disappointed by your mistakes. Simply notice, *Okay, I've made a mistake. It's completely human, and potentially helpful.* For what? For your learning process. Now you're going to ask, *All right. I didn't do something the way I should have done it, but what is my lesson?* Remember that there is a lesson in everything we do wrong, and there is a lesson in every crisis. If you learn the lesson of your crisis, of your pain, your disease process, your relationships, your friendships, and even the lessons of your own aging process, then you're not going to make the same mistakes again. Learning the lessons of your mistakes is a matter of determination, of self-actualizing. Actualize your intent. *My intent is not to make the same mistake twice.* Change the way you do business.

We all have many experiences in life, but they do not guarantee growth. If you know how to extract the lesson from an experience, then every experience is potentially a growth process. How many times do we do things just because we're up for doing them or we're in a place to do them, but they yield no lessons? You can have thousands of experiences and learn nothing from them unless you remember to ask, "What is the lesson of this experience?" Let the experience work for you.

I find that most people have outgrown their lives. They have outgrown many of their friendships, and in some cases they have outgrown other relationships as well. Many people are living too small a life, and feel as frustrated and uncomfortable as if they were wearing clothes so tight that they can't breathe, but they don't want to change their clothing. Don't be afraid to expand your consciousness to the size of your life. We tend to just accept the size of the life we've been given, and adjust to it rather than transcend the expectations of others to live the life we want to live.

Everything is in motion, so be okay wherever you are. My first apartment in Manhattan was a unique little place: one room with a bathtub in the kitchen. My bathtub was opposite my kitchen sink, and it was such a tiny bathtub that I had to scrunch way up to get into it, and had to pour a pot water over myself to get washed, but rent was $57 a month, and that was all I could afford. *This is okay for now,* I told myself, and I remember being pleased because I knew it was just a transition.

Everything in life is in motion, I realized, *so this is just a moment in time. I'm in one situation that is moving, which will take me to another place (preferably with a larger tub).* Why be angry about where you're at? That's like being impatient when you're in first grade because you want to be in tenth grade. Be patient, because if you keep a steady eye on what you must do and you allow your life to open up, gradually your expectations, perceptions, vision, and ideals mature until one day you're like an eagle whose wings are spread and can finally soar.

Without patience you may settle for a very limited sense of who you are and a very narrow sense of the world you're in. You may shut yourself down by living a restricted life with very little understanding of the larger picture. You may see only the surface of things, never looking deeply, in contrast to those who patiently transcend superficiality and selfishness to enjoy a profound appreciation of life.

So be okay where you are—for now. Decide, *It's okay that I'm overweight, temporarily. It's okay that I'm fatigued, because the process that I've chosen for myself is going to take me to where I should be. And when I get there, I'll create a whole new ideal, and I'll open up another door as well.* And then one day, like that youthful woman in her seventies winning a national championship, you will have fulfilled much of your potential. That woman was so fit for her age that seeing all the other seventy-year-olds lined up beside her, you would think she was in the wrong row. Now how about deciding that you don't have to remain forever in the row you're in? Choose the one where you'd like to be.

Expand your awareness of your life, and your life expands with it. Break out of the mold and be yourself. Open up and expand instead of impersonating your notion of what you think the world expects you to be. If you expand your awareness of your life, your life will expand with all of its potential. You are the only one who is holding you back. Don't blame others, and certainly don't blame circumstances.

Where in your life are you frustrated? Where do you have intractable conflict? Causes are important. The anti-war movement and the human rights movement are legitimate. Just don't become a casualty of your own zeal and lose your authentic self because of it. The only reason I've been able to be a part of so many causes for so long and have helped so many movements along is because I don't wake up every morning and say, *My God, my life is worthless because I've spent eight years on this cause and nothing has happened.* I don't want to feel bad about myself because I can't convince other people out there to make changes. I wake up every morning and say, *My life is great.* Yes, there are things that have got to be done in this world, but I'm still going to maintain my positive attitude no matter what happens out there. You don't have to make an excuse for that.

Be the supportive, enthusiastic person who is an example of someone who stands for something from a place of positive energy, rather than the person who is disheveled emotionally, spiritually, and psychically. So many activists are spent, reduced to going through the motions of fighting, fighting, and more fighting, as if the main thing in life were conflict, not realizing that love is a greater conqueror than fear and hate. One day they wake up filled with as much hate as the people they're against who are filled with hate. Hate is hate, fear is fear; anger is anger, destructive energy is destructive energy, no matter which side of a cause it comes from. Intractable conflict occurs when people who have joined a movement lose their sense of self in the cause, forgetting their humanity and getting caught in the machinery of hating their opponents.

Take a careful look at the many movements with leaders and members who are angry, burnt out, and bitter. They are highly reactionary, having lost touch with their spiritual side. Then think of someone like Gandhi or Martin Luther King, Jr., who never lost his joy and respect for life, including regard for the lives of those who held contrary views. I remember being in a peace march during the Vietnam War, and as we marched down the street, people around me were screaming that they wished the war supporters on the sidelines would be killed. I said, "Then what differentiates you from them? How are you different from the war supporter if you want someone killed and he wants someone killed?"

Cultivate patience or you will lose your balance. One of my buddies gave up his relationship with his family because he could not control the anger that he held from the movement when he came home at night. Uncertain of the progress of his cause, he'd yell at his relatives, and once, when his wife suggested that they go out to a movie, he became violent and smacked her because she wasn't a true comrade of the cause. Look at what that does to your kids. It can get so easy for people to be self-righteous to justify their inexcusable behavior.

Support a worthy cause, but support your life at the same time. Keep your emotional balance. Enjoy your relationships and each day wake up and be thankful that you have another day to live. Detach from the outcome of your efforts because if you don't, when something fails you'll go right down the hole with it. Then you've got a double problem: You've got a cause that is wearing you out because you feel helpless and impotent to do anything about it, and then you become angry and despondent and complain with other angry, despondent people. Support causes, but support them realizing that all causes take much time and energy, and they may not change in your lifetime. Do not give up your life and the joys of your lifetime because of the cause. I've seen too many people do that.

Where are you going to find the truth? What if you were to demand a higher standard of truth? Almost all of your illusions would be swept away. What happens when you believe in illusion, but imagine you have the truth? You can't question it. You're not willing to because it's dogma. You react angrily if anyone challenges you. What causes that anger? You feel defensive. You feel threatened that someone may take away what you feel confident and comfortable with. So if you want to find the truth, you must first detect the illusions you support. Are you working for a standard of living or a quality of life? If everyone wanted to work for a better quality of life, most of us would have to change our jobs. You might have to change where you live to cut the commute to make time for your family.

What happens when you start to separate yourself from all illusions? First you are disappointed that you trusted in things that were illusory, and aren't certain what to believe anymore. But as you progress, you begin to see real truths, and then you begin to respect those real truths a few at a time. Eventually you discover that the truth is easy. Maintaining illusion is what's really difficult. Illusion requires reinforcing lies and deceptions to sustain dogmas and rituals as if they had real meaning and substance. We're afraid to pull back the curtain to see that the Wizard of Oz is our illusion.

Ask yourself what is more expensive: embracing the truth to be healthy or holding yourself captive in the illusion of normalcy by supersizing everything and buying products you don't need because stars endorse them on TV? Obesity and debt, now considered to be American epidemics, are high prices to pay to stay in our trance of illusion.

Look at the Wall Street mogul. Look at corporate America where all too frequently there's another scandal. Regularly major corporations are found guilty of earning enormous amounts of money through unethical means. Why do they need more? Why would a person who already makes ten or one hundred million dollars a year need more money? Because no matter how much money they make they never feel authentic. They never feel complete. They never feel whole. They never feel truly connected to what is important to them. Life's true rewards are found by those who are the most loving. You're going to remember the person who gave you exceptional moments. The exceptional moments are joy, happiness, humor, and love, right? That's the person you want to be around. You don't want to be around people who are greedy, selfish, and conceited, no matter what they're worth. And yet they don't understand that. So they'll go out tonight instead of being home with the family to continue to make deals because they don't know when enough is enough. They don't know when to stop. We're talking ten million Americans who don't know when they have enough and just can't appreciate what they have.

Do you choose to limit your opportunities? How do you choose to limit yourself? You might assume that circumstances or others limit you, but I suggest that you tend to limit yourself by not believing in your completeness. When you accept that you are complete, that you have everything you need in order to achieve anything you choose, you will find that you can connect with other people simply by sharing that positive energy, and your limitations disappear.

Does fear hold you back? Stop struggling with life. Do you assume the role of victim, as many people do, because you don't seem to have enough? Perhaps you don't think you have enough money or contacts, or you don't have the right looks, or something is missing; so you hold yourself back with the fear that if you try to do something, you may fail. But it is your very fear of failure, your fear of being ridiculed and humiliated, and of losing your self-esteem, that prevents you from moving ahead.

Live smoothly: create an ease of living, an ease of thinking, and an ease of being. Make an honest effort, but don't struggle. Watch how great athletes run so effortlessly, so smoothly. Live your life that way. When you're at ease, you're not in disease. When we shock and overstress ourselves, we're left with the consequences—disease. The very thing we're after, good health through balance, is denied us. Stop struggling with everything. Life is not meant to be an obstacle course. It's more like school. Trust in life's generosity as your teacher.

We are a society that thinks the more we multitask the more we achieve. Nothing could be farther from the truth. Multitasking is not a synonym for accomplishment. It's better to do a few things well in balance than to multitask and start failing. Think of all the things we juggle in a day, and with every extra task that we toss in there's a greater chance for things to go wrong, until one day all we're doing is struggling to keep our balance, nothing more. We're no longer able to appreciate what we do because we've lost contact with who we are. We fall out of touch with the importance of our mission. We have no sensitivity left to be able to feel anything. We're overwhelmed to the point of being numb.

Start to delegate your optional responsibilities. Make a list of the things you will no longer do, both inside and outside of your home, and then explain to others that in order to reclaim your life and protect your family, you must stop overcommitting yourself. It may take three or four months before you actually feel comfortable after you stop multitasking. You're like someone who's trying to give up caffeine after you've been drinking ten cups a day; you're not going to stop and then feel good right away. You're going to go through multitasking withdrawal but that's all right, because for every moment that you reclaim, you're regaining the most precious asset you have—your time.

Do you realize how much of your time you lose to your tasks? At the end of the day are you better because of it? Is the world a better place because of it? Is your relationship better for it? So start disengaging from your excess responsibilities now. Don't give that time away. Give it back to yourself, and then look at what you could do. Go to museums. Go see the botanical gardens. Spend time with people you love. They deserve your time. That is never time wasted because it is part of reconnecting with the essential.

You already know your life's mission. Every cell in your body has its mission, its knowledge of what to do cooperatively. To say that your body is a well-coordinated system to support life is an understatement. Trust in the unlimited wisdom of that life. All you need to do is to get quiet, be at peace, at ease, and the distinctive picture of your life will reveal itself—because you already know it.

One day you will realize, *My goodness, all this was right in front of me. Why didn't I see it?* The camouflage of clutter, busyness, and too much responsibility breeds anxieties, fears, and judgments that can distort your reality. Stop searching for meaning and purpose through a fog of illusion. Discover which of your beliefs have brought you to worship your mountain of shallow tasks, surplus property,

and poisons, and then disengage from them to discover your freedom. Unburden yourself. Stop overdoing the inessentials. When you
reconnect with what is essential and reinstate balance in your life,
you will see that you have a restorative prescription for your soul
because you are honoring it.

CHAPTER FIFTEEN

Being Present for Your Own Life

What does it mean to be present for your own life? Most of us try diligently to maintain a sense of identity, which we do by establishing some order, setting certain boundaries, and keeping our thoughts and actions in line with our conditioning, in order to be acceptable to society. Why not? We all want to be accepted, but it's better to be accepted and appreciated for who you truly are than to be a poor example of what others think you should be.

Your constructed "self" is an illusion. Illusion often enters into the mix when you think you are only as valuable as your credit card, your employee ID, or your mate. We even tend to identify ourselves with our pets. Props such as these (and for some, they are props) become an extension of what one thinks of as a self. These may all be perceived as parts of who "I" am.

So how do we start discerning who we really are, and become present to the truth of our lives? The only way you can be present is to stop constantly looking over your shoulder to see whether or not you are doing everything right. That distraction is an easy way to remain oblivious to your life. Are you just going through the motions of your life without even knowing what they are? Everything you keep referring to from your past could be misaligned. Some of your beliefs and values could be wrong. If so, then everything you are going to do in this moment will be from a mistaken viewpoint; you will feel a sense of *why me?* when anything goes wrong. When we were young we couldn't understand either intellectually or viscerally that our conditioned responses were self-defeating. We just did what was expected of us because there was reward if we obeyed and punishment if we didn't. Still today, if you follow society's dictates, you'll be rewarded, even if what you're asked to do is immoral. You have to do as you are told. If you challenge prevailing ideas, then you're considered wrong and you're punished.

First, pay attention to what is going on. Instead of worrying about all of society's ills, start your journey with yourself. Ask if what you contribute to the world is constructive and authentic or destructive. When other people become objects for your use, you become a puppeteer, pulling as many strings as possible; a master manipulator. You fail to see anything that does not serve your narrow purposes of satisfaction. You can't truly evaluate what you're doing until you slow down long enough to be fully present.

My generation, the baby boomers, has mastered the art of hyperspeed. We're overly fast at everything. We want everything instantly. We are the headline generation. They call it "hurry disease"—people glancing at their watches constantly, pulling their dog's leash before he's finished his business, letting their children trail far behind them as they go rushing forth on the city streets or in department stores. We used to call this "impatience," and that's just what it is. You can call it a fancy disease, but it's still impatience, plain and simple. And it comes without awareness. It's automatic. To stop you must catch yourself at it and see that it is ugly. The patience and determination to understand life is frequently lost in the frantic process of juggling many speedy tasks. You have to go deeper than that to find substance.

More often than not, when we are thrown a curve ball in life, we respond first by feeling helpless with acute anxiety. We don't know how to handle all those balls going into the air. We're afraid of dropping them. There comes a point in life when you simply have to step back and let everything go.

Watch how the leaves gracefully spiral and drift from their branches in the fall. That's what they are made to do; they allow the wind to carry them where it will. They never try to cling desperately to their branch, as we do in life. Their beauty goes on, as they continue giving to the earth.

Let everything in your life simply cease to be significant for a moment. What happens when you do that? Your breathing becomes more relaxed. You may smile. You suddenly become aware in that moment that you have a moment.

In the rush to get things done, we fail to think of the consequences of our words upon others, to consider how what we've said might impact another human being. Was I gracious and humble or sarcastic and demeaning? Was I supportive or sharp, encouraging or critical? How you are feeling about yourself directly impacts how you feel about others. We often see that when Mom reprimands little Jennifer, Jennifer turns around and scolds her dolly, or her baby sister or Fido. It's a trickledown effect. If you don't feel good about yourself, you're not apt to like others. And we do tend to copy other people's actions and attitudes.

If you don't feel good about yourself or others, you may view anyone else who feels good about themselves as a threat. There's not a real threat there. You just think there is. One person's happiness does not in any way undermine another's, but we're overly competitive, so to be charitable and respect other people by supporting their success feels like we're helping the enemy. When you look at this generation, not that it's unique or exclusive to us, but one of the things you notice is that we don't spend a lot of time looking at the consequences of our actions.

When I was in high school, all five thousand of us students went through school liking some teachers, disliking others, but we all had something in common: respect for our teachers. That school was a proving ground for developing our character and our sense of social responsibility.

If someone threw something on the ground, I can promise you someone else would say, "Pick it up. It doesn't belong there." If you were a pregnant woman or a senior citizen and you got on a bus, someone would immediately give you his or her seat. Go on a subway today and watch a teenage boy or girl race a pregnant woman or a senior citizen to a seat. Just sitting comfortably while a pregnant woman or a senior citizen or a disabled person stands right in front of you means you are indifferent to others. This is the opposite of being present for your life.

Watch people throw garbage onto the streets of New York City without any concern because no one's going to say anything to them. As I walk past Manhattan skyscrapers, I see employees thoughtlessly throw away their cigarettes toward passersby, as if to blame us for the law that sends them outdoors to smoke. I have seen people toss their lit cigarettes onto the upscale streets of Boston from their balconies, and saw students throw a large wooden desk out of a fourth-floor window of a Boston tenement. We have lost respect for our fellow human beings.

Treating others with dignity and respect and being able to disagree courteously means that you are maturely in charge of your own life. Character development and moral guidance must be nurtured in the home and encouraged by society so that we will treat each other with dignity and respect. You don't have to attack a person to challenge their ideas. Even if you disagree with someone, learn to differ with respect.

I'm going to raise some ideas and questions here to help you think about how present you are in different areas of your life, and what choices you make, and why. Spend time with them. You could spend at least an hour focusing on any one of them. Take a quiet, meditative moment to contemplate those that speak to you the most.

Break through your drab routines. Try something new and evaluate it. What is the significance of the experience? All of our experiences have significance. They may not all be life-changing, but every single experience contains a message. Your new experience can be something as simple as trying a different restaurant and a different type of food. You could try going to a market where you've never shopped and buying something you haven't bought before. You might read a book that is different from any you've read before. Try changing your routines throughout a day. Or open yourself up to new friendships to see if there are people of different backgrounds, ages, and genders with whom you could associate. Something wonderful happens when we start making new connections that feel right, but we often have to break a pattern to discover them.

Evaluate your friends. Do you know how dependable they really are? A real friend is there whether you are going through thick or through thin. They are there at the bottom and not just at the top. It's easy to say you're a friend when there's no challenge. It's a different story when there are hard times.

Do you learn from the mistakes and weaknesses of others? You can learn from other's weaknesses even if they can't see their own. If someone is dishonest, you learn about the significance of dishonesty, and if that trait is in you at any level you can examine it. You can notice the ways you're being dishonest and can correct yourself.

What experiences do you avoid because you're afraid of the consequences? What, specifically, are you afraid of? Some experiences that people avoid, although they could really only help, include: exercising, eating right, meditation, seeing the world, and introducing themselves to other cultures, people, and their values.

Is everything you've been taught to trust limited to one bound book or one neighborhood or one family or one medical system? If so, you could feel threatened by anything that challenges what you were told about the safety of your bounded experience. The trouble with a bounded existence is that you're told what to believe, how to believe, how to live, and that everything you've ever questioned can be answered from a very limited perspective.

When your bounded existence proves too small and fails you, do you panic and attempt to run away in your mind? Imagine what happens when, one day, you wake up in a crisis and you find that the tools you were given don't work. You are disempowered. You feel anxious. At the point of acute anxiety, people start making really foolish decisions. That's when we start doing self-destructive things: gambling, overeating, taking drugs, overworking, hiding, denying, and going a mile a minute. We do anything to keep from feeling. So in effect, we put life into distraction mode.

Are you in a relationship to distract yourself from your life? If so, instead of growing in maturity, you may be abdicating responsibility for your life. One of the best ways in the world to distract yourself is to be in a relationship, especially a bad one. It's not that relationships are bad. They're not, but if the reason you are in a relationship is to distract yourself, then it's not a good relationship. You will tend to be with very immature types; either a screaming, jealous, possibly violent dominator or someone who constantly needs your help with decisions, including finances, as would a child. Anyone who disrupts your peace keeps you from being present for your own life and growing. Can you see how you chose that person so you could run away from reality into a chaos of your own making? There is a story of a woman walking a long distance who sees a wounded snake by the roadside, feels sorry for him, and picks him up, seeking companionship, stimulation, and appreciation for her kindness. After a mile, the snake bit the woman. "Why did you bite me?" asked the woman before the venom killed her, "I was good to you." The snake answered, "You knew I was a viper when you picked me up."

Do you procrastinate to avoid life? We become chronic procrastinators. We work around problems, but never face them. You must face a problem for what it is if you want to change. You have to look it right in the eye and not blink, and realize there's nothing to be afraid of.

Do you make decisions based on your own observations or did someone tell you the right thing to do? Think of how many times you've wasted money on something or kept someone in your life just because it was considered the right thing to do. Right by whose standards?

The people who created the box that you've been placed in? Then one day, whether you're a woman or black or Latino or a senior citizen or rich or poor or middle class or you live on the East Coast or the West Coast or in Middle America, you no longer have any identity. You're simply a consumer. After all, isn't that what we're called? Now consumers do what? They consume. Which means they do what? Buy. Now people who consume are economic what? Indicators. Yes. Well, there's another word not quite as polite—slaves.

Do you evaluate people by how famous they are or by how many degrees they have instead of by your own experience with them? Do you discriminate between Ivy League schools and others? If you don't have a degree and someone else does, then you're not considered as smart as the person who has the degree. Remember that in *The Wizard of Oz,* the Wizard gives the Scarecrow an honorary ThD, Doctor of Thinkology diploma, to prove that he has a brain; and the Cowardly Lion is awarded the Courage Medal to show that he is brave. We only feel that we're somebody if we have something that says so.

Everywhere you look someone's trying to tell you that you're not good enough or smart enough or pretty enough or happy enough or strong enough or healthy enough or intelligent enough or successful enough on your own. Only by following them and giving to them will you ever be acceptable. They have to create the illusion and then sell it to you. You have to buy into it and once you buy into it, you're committed. Now they've got you.

Approval-seeking halts your progress. If you feel confident in yourself only by proving something to others, then you will remain caught in the cycle of doing things for other people instead of for yourself. You should never live for other people's approval, whether it's about the size of your house, the style of your clothes, money in the bank, or anything else. Then you're not a human being of free will, but a puppet of someone else's expectations.

What would change if you stop this need to be someplace else, with someone else, doing something else, because you're really not content or happy with what you are now? What would change is freeing up all that energy you're putting into the wrong area. We haven't learned how to go inside; we're always externalizing. How do you think we end up spending more money than we make and end up with credit card debt higher than it has ever been? Do we really need everything that we buy? No. We don't. But we think we do.

Something urges you to reach into your pocket to get that credit card. *I need this.* What if there was some kind of behavioralist there at the checkout counter to ask you, "Why are you buying this? You already have a pair of jeans. You don't need another pair of Levi's. Now think before you buy it." You'd say, "I do have three pairs of jeans. So what's another one?" or, "Well, I just felt like buying them." "Why? How are you going to pay for them?" Wouldn't it be great if there was someone to talk us out of every sale, or even to assail us on the road? "Why are you talking on the cell phone while driving? Is that call so important?" "No. It's not."

Why is there no one to help us at the checkout counter or to save us on the road or to help us whenever there's a choice to be made? The answer is that there would be no need for you to be present for your own life if you had a guardian of the sort I've just presented. You need to become self-reliant in order to grow and mature. You must be alert to ask yourself the questions that will help you find balance in each situation. If Jeeves were always there with you, prompting you, you would become dependent on him and never find out who you are.

When we feel out of control in our lives, we tend to make choices that cloud our perception in subtle ways. When you are upset, for example, you may overeat, and the choice to binge may give you a sugar high that boosts your mood, but only temporarily; then you are worse off when your comfort fades and you feel the full weight of the issue you were avoiding. You need to get a clear perspective on what is happening in your life, even if what you end up seeing is ugly. I'd rather see an ugly picture that's honest than an artificial picture that is temporary and deceptive.

Every experience can be a lesson for us: a good lesson, a bad lesson, a positive lesson, a painful lesson, or a joyful lesson. Whatever we ultimately want to do with the experience, at least it can teach us something. It's how many times we keep making the same mistake that becomes the problem. The accumulation of mistakes wears us down.

How much better it would be if we only made a mistake once in a given area and learned from it so we didn't have to make it again. But we are serial repeaters. We make all these mistakes over and over again. So we have to ask, *What experience do I choose to bring into my life today to allow me to be more present to my life?* That way you can say, *Well, I liked it or I didn't like it, but at least I didn't stop myself from experiencing it.* With practice you move beyond all of your conditioned responses that say you shouldn't even have a particular experience.

Whatever you do, be present in the moment and judge it in the moment. Judge it for what it is, and not for what you thought it would be or was told it would be. That's how we break down barriers of all kinds. Talk with someone from another race and be present for that conversation. Let it be what it is. If you don't, then you will always have the assumption that somehow you shouldn't be in that conversation; or you shouldn't be traveling to that place, shouldn't be eating that food, shouldn't be engaging in that activity.

What is awakened awareness? Awakened awareness is completely being in the moment I'm in right now. I don't need anything from my past to be aware that I am thinking and breathing. Just be centered. It's a living meditation, so every moment of every day you're not missing anything.

If you walk through a garden, you're present in the garden. You see the butterflies. You hear the hummingbird. You see the bees. You see the bugs crawling. You can smell the aromas because you're present for them. You're awakening yourself. It's as if your mind opens up and this wonderful rose blooms. That's what it means to be awakening. Right now, many of us are not awake. We're asleep. We're in a stupor. Why? Because it's uncomfortable to awaken. We don't want to go through the pain of awakening because all of our illusions will be reexamined. Once you're awakened, you don't want to live by illusions anymore. Reality is far richer and more interesting than any illusion.

Experience things by being awake and present for them. The moment you reach back to the past, you're not awakened in the moment. Look at life nonjudgmentally by being present for it. Otherwise, you're going to judge everything. We do judge everything, but for a moment go to neutral, look honestly at what you're judging, then decide what judgment you should offer. This prevents you from merely reacting, and so lessens the conditioned mind's input.

Rest, repair, and visualize before your journey. We don't give ourselves an opportunity to start life correctly. When you watch runners before a race, you never see them just jump out of a car and start to run. They stretch and relax and ease into motion. Before I run a race, I visualize the entire race. I visualize how I want to do it and how I'm going to feel. Then when I'm in the race, I'm simply present for the energy in each moment. I'm not thinking of anything else. My mind is not distracted. It's like a laser. I'm focused, but before that, I had to be rested. I couldn't have my mind cluttered with all kinds of thoughts. That's why you have to separate out what's real in the now from all the thoughts you can't control.

What you can't control is what clutters your mind. What you keep obsessing about is not what you've done that you enjoy, but what you can't control, what isn't working, what is troubling you, and what is challenging. You keep revisiting thoughts over and over and over again in your mind because that's the only place where you have some control over the outcome. It's either excuses or justifications; none of that is positive.

When you let go of your relentless thinking, you can rest. Once you're relaxed, visualize what you want and start your journey. When we wake up we just jump into the day. We're so focused on starting our rituals and routine that we don't visualize the greater importance of the day. This is a twenty-four-hour period we can never live again. So what can we do in this twenty-four hours that's new and unique, empowering and fulfilling?

We can keep ourselves challenged and alert even in the small details of our lives. Every dinner I make is original. I never prepare exactly the same dinner twice. I even vary the health drinks I make each time, throwing in a different fruit, using rice milk instead of soymilk. We start getting old mentally when we no longer look to enrich ourselves with a challenging environment. If you take it easy and settle for work or a relationship that is comfortable, you get in a rut. Then one day, you've gone from enrichment to boredom, to tediousness and indifference, and you become apathetic and depressed.

We all have emotional minefields that can easily be triggered. Someone sets us off and we react. We go out to the diner and order more food than we need or buy a quart of ice cream, smoke marijuana, or drink alcohol, or something else that's not good for our health. Some are stoned on drugs or tranquilizers, others on their own needs. Some people do meditation not because it is freeing, but because they find it calming and adaptive. They lead very hectic and stressed lives, and they meditate because they can feel very blissful and detached from their pain. Or they practice their yoga, getting right into it, and then go outside and smoke a cigarette and get on the cell phone and start yelling. Then meditation or yoga becomes an escape in the same way that we use cocaine or heroin or marijuana. No different from a pound of chocolate cake. It's a distraction. Now if they use meditation as a way of transforming themselves, that's different. Otherwise, it's just an escape without ingesting chemicals.

If the only way you feel alive is to feel some emotion, then you're going to draw that energy to you. You'll be the drama queen, where every thing is a drama. Or you'll be the needy queen. When we get stuck in these roles, we can go on automatic. Someone can actually predict what you're going to say, how you're going to say it, and the way you're going to feel. You can see these patterns in people you know. You know what they're going to say and how they're going to respond even before you talk. That means you're just a set of emotions.

Seeking can also be a distraction from our own dramas. I know many people who run around the world seeking. What is it out there we're seeking? Are we going to run off to India and meditate with a guru? Will that give us our identity? Our journey is here. No matter where you take yourself, you're still with yourself. So if you're insecure here, you're going to be insecure wherever you go. Whomever you're with, you're still going to be the same person. We like to think that we're going to be different with a different person, but we're not. We'd have to transform ourselves to be different.

So we do a lot of running and a lot of hiding, just so we can feel better about ourselves. Then we start dreaming. *If only I had a better job, a different place to live, a kinder person to be with, then I would feel better about myself.* It doesn't work—I've never seen anyone who improved because they got what they thought they needed. If you feel incomplete now, you're going to feel incomplete no matter whom you're with or what circumstances you're in as long as you keep chasing externals instead of doing the internal work that's necessary for real change.

Did it ever occur to you that responsibility for yourself starts with just you? We need to make it a solo process. I encourage you to take the time to experience the pain that leads to accepting who you are, with your weaknesses and strengths completely revealed, and then focus on detaching and transcending through understanding and surrender. So when you go out in the world, you go as a whole person with a fresh mind, and not out of need. It's better to have a complete sense of self.

You have to change your perspective to change your conditioning. That's a test you must give yourself. Do you have the courage to deconstruct all these illusions by which you live, about what you need or who you are, how you should look and how you should be, how you should act around other people, and how you should be affected?

Only when you can take that step, and it's a courageous step, to challenge yourself, to test yourself, and learn whether you pass or fail the test, will you be present for your own life. It's okay to fail the test as long as you learn why you failed and then reapply that to the next lesson of life. Then our failure on one test becomes the lesson that we must learn. Then one day you don't fail that test because you've learned the lesson.

Think of yourself at your best, at your strongest, your happiest, your most effervescent, and at your most dynamic and passionate. That's where you should direct your energy and where your visions of self should come from because you realize that you're capable of all of that growth.

What are the tools you need to get there? Patience. Determination. Discipline. Respect. Compassion. Belief. Believe in the moment. If you place your faith in the moment, you are free from limitation. Instead of giving your power to everyone else, you can take back some power for yourself.

Some years ago, I ran into an eighty-one-year-old woman who lived in my apartment building at a supermarket. She had two gallons of milk and a cheesecake in her cart. "Oh, I listen to you all the time, have for years," she said. I didn't ask her about her purchases. She was one of those people whose behavior did not appear to agree with her own better judgment.

She stopped to chat and before long, she was telling me how her father had refused to let her go to art school when she was a teenager. To that very day, she still resented her father for depriving her of art school over sixty years ago. I asked, "Did you have time for art school after your children grew up?" "Yes," she said. "Why didn't you go?" I asked. "Oh, my father would not have approved had he been alive." That meant that she was forbidden from ever following her dream of art. Probably, prisoner of the past that she was, she did not allow herself to pursue other interests either. There was a pattern of futility to which she had assented throughout her life. Oh, why bother to try to actually do anything, whether it be art or change of diet? That is what happens when we are absent from our own life and true needs.

That's no way to live. We need to start living with a simple process of inner awareness and being present in this moment. Remember, every day is a good day.

CHAPTER SIXTEEN

Now or Never

Benjamin Franklin astutely observed that you can be certain of nothing in life except death and taxes. He neglected to include perhaps the most inexorable of all life's conditions—crisis. From the most powerful tycoon on Wall Street to the most deprived supplicant in Bangladesh, crisis will strike at some point. For some it takes the form of a tragic death in the family. For others, severe financial setbacks or the loss of a long-held job are extreme crises which must be faced. For many, crisis will appear as a sudden injury or a major health catastrophe such as a stroke. The list can be endless. But I believe the key that can have a profound effect on our response and offer a whole new positive approach and appreciation for life is how we define crisis itself.

Let's take stroke as an example of crisis. It is the third leading cause of death in the United States behind heart disease and cancer. Consider what it would be like to suffer a stroke and be lucky enough to survive. How would you react, coming so close to losing all the aspects of life you hold so dear? All of a sudden your family, friends, and pets are seen in a whole new light. The places you love going, the foods you love eating, and the activities you love doing are no longer taken for granted. In this way the crisis becomes your gift. Yesterday's distractions become today's insignificances. You realize that you failed to pay attention to your real needs and thus created the imbalances that set the stage for a stroke in the first place. The same pattern of imbalance applies to the crisis of cancer, heart attack, obesity, or any relationship or financial crisis. They are all a process; an accumulation of many, many choices. Crisis is the universe's way of guiding us back to balance.

Now, most people will look at events such as these and label them tragedies. They may retreat and be afraid to do anything. But the crisis is part of our life journey and is meant to teach and assist us. Everything and everyone in our lives—the good, the bad, the pleasurable, and the terrible—are all there to help us along the journey. If we pay attention to that assistance, we can learn from it. We can learn that like a game of chess, every thought and action in life has a consequence.

Unfortunately, most people view crisis through a prism of fear. Fear constricts. It constricts your body and your mind. When the mind constricts it fears taking chances and when enough behavior becomes conditioned to avoid taking chances, growth ceases and fear wins. The cycle of avoidance spreads into other areas of our lives and pretty soon we stop trying anything new or different to avoid being criticized, laughed at, or simply thought of as different. Staying safe and comfortable becomes the modus operandi, and risk aversion the primary purpose. The problem is, this living in fear of change leads to stagnation and grave imbalance. Crisis is the universe warning us to make necessary course corrections on our journey through life. You will find that the great crises that happen in people's lives are usually preceded by earlier promptings for change that went unheeded. Crisis is the universe's way of getting you to listen.

Look at your life and ask yourself what is it that you are not paying attention to. What ideas have you abrogated responsibility for, allowing some pseudo-authority figure who really doesn't have your best interests at heart to make your decisions? Nobody knows you like you know yourself. The Oracle at Delphi—an enduring pinnacle of wisdom for Western civilization—stipulated only two things: "Know thyself," and "Nothing in excess." If you know yourself and take charge consciously of making choices that serve you and your growth, your life will achieve a balance, and in that balance will come a harmony and a healthy life force that will not be creating crisis, for you will live every day in direct connection with your vital, true self.

If you are overweight, you haven't been paying attention. If your spouse wants a divorce, you haven't been paying attention. As with our example of a stroke, any life events we label "crisis" follow the same pattern. Being unhealthy requires the same commitment as being healthy. A lot of energy goes into making the wrong choices day in and day out over time. Hundreds of thousands of incorrectly chosen mouthfuls of food, and thousands of days of denial about the necessity of exercise go into making a person obese. The underlying motivations take the same consistency of effort that a marathon runner exhibits, only in reverse. It takes the same energy and the same time commitment; the same rules apply. Every effect has a cause, and the same cause repeated over and over yields a consistent effect.

If you're overweight, think how you got there. Examine why you continued to make choices that you knew were going to cause this negative outcome. It's not an accident, but intentional self-sabotage. It's intentional because you have to give the wrong path time, commitment, and energy. You have to give it emotion and a myriad of complex defense mechanisms to justify what you're doing. The ego justifies the bad mistake you're making.

Let's say you lost your job after twenty years. Naturally you would feel unappreciated and slighted that something like that would happen to you after all those years of sacrifice. If you had been let go sooner, you would have been growing in other ways and learned that in the end the job was simply a way of allowing you to go on to the next step in your life. The opportunity can be a great gift to allow you to grow on your own.

We generally do things we know we won't fail at. This fear of failure turns people into robots, doing the same things the same way, day in and day out. It takes a lot of courage to do something you don't know how to do. In all likelihood it will take repeated effort to get better at that something, but that's what makes life exciting and interesting. Look at yourself as a renaissance person—trying everything, experimenting, experiencing. When you're no longer attached you can do anything because you don't have to worry whether you win or lose. You don't have to care if you do it right or wrong because the process of doing is what matters and what honors life. When you reach that point you can do anything. Too often we distract ourselves instead of focusing. When we start a project we'll look for something to distract us—the television, the radio, the phone, food—anything to occupy our time, to avoid the diligence and patience necessary to master that project. When you're distracted you can't focus, and when you can't focus you don't have presence of mind in the moment. In order to grow you must put an end to distractions and learn to focus. You have to be conscious in the moment, and then you have to create balance in that moment. The only way to get healthy and conquer self-sabotage and the incompleteness in our lives is to figure out where we have allowed imbalance into our lives. When you wake up each day you have twenty-four hours of time. Focusing more time for work than play will cause an imbalance. That imbalance will cause stress, which then leads to distress that then leads to hormonal and blood sugar imbalances. These lead to local inflammatory conditions and pains, which lead to neurological damage and premature aging, all because of trying to do too much work in a given day. Give the appropriate amount of time necessary in each area of your life every day, and balance and growth, progress and achievement will be yours.

We often forget that play is an absolute must each and every day. Albert Einstein said that if he couldn't play his violin every day he couldn't think as well. Choose the play that gives you joy and happiness. Don't play based upon what someone else says is the right play, but play what you want to play. Don't eat because it's mealtime, but eat when your body is hungry; that's when your body needs nutrients. Don't eat everything on your plate just because it's there. That will lead to you being overweight. Don't rush and distract yourself with things like television while you eat. Take your time and enjoy the taste of the food. Reorganize your day if you need to so that no one tells you that your work is more important than your nourishment.

Instead of enjoying our food we're usually concerned about the next thing that needs to be done. We keep looking to the future instead of focusing on where we are or what we are doing. This distraction creates imbalance; imbalance affects digestion and energy doesn't get really to where it needs to go. Slow down, create a meal that honors your body, and turn off the cell phone and TV. Put away your magazines and savor the experience of eating.

When you set up time to play don't let work interfere. More and more people bring their work with them on vacation, spending time on their cell phones and their laptops. Others play too hard while on vacation; too much play can result in imbalance as well. They don't spend time resting and relaxing, and by the end of vacation are exhausted and almost glad to be back. Too frequently people are driven to be in a constant state of activity to the point where they can't just sit back and relax. There is a time for work, play, rest, and relaxation.

We also have to learn how to make time for ourselves. Oftentimes in relationships we're made to feel guilty because we need our space. We may watch a ballgame, a television program, spend time with our friends, or any number of things that we may enjoy to which our partner objects. Suddenly there is guilt and shame for the time we are spending on ourselves. Create space for yourself and don't apologize for it. Don't ask for it as though you were a slave asking permission of a benevolent master. It's your life and you need to establish your rules and boundaries. The first rule is that you're important. Other people in your life are important too, but they must acknowledge your time, needs, and energy. When you establish those boundaries you no longer have the stress that occurs when you're trying to serve everyone else's needs and neglecting your own.

Feeling guilty that you're not doing enough, you may spend all your energy doing things for other people. This creates an imbalance in your life. Instead, start the day as the center of your own life, and let everything emanate from that beginning. If you're healthy and balanced, everyone will benefit from that positive energy. If you're unhealthy and unbalanced, no one will benefit. Putting yourself first is often called selfish, but it's self-love. There is a big difference between the two.

When you eat, when you sleep, when you play, when you're engaged in your hobbies, whatever else you do, make sure that the day has balance. Turn off the television. Do something that challenges the mind and creates intellectual balance. Start a creative project that stretches the mind and forces it to think and thus grow and develop. That's healthy and important. Remember the Greek ideal of balance between mind, body, and spirit. Attention to each facet of yourself leads to a greater understanding of yourself as a complete being.

Disease doesn't easily manifest in the existence of balance. A healthy diet contains the nutrients to keep your blood thin—vitamin E, vitamin C, magnesium—are all natural blood thinners. You have the energy that your body needs for your brain to think, and your body to repair itself and to rejuvenate. You're able to take in the proper nutrients because you've given yourself the time to prepare and assimilate a healthy diet. Every single action has a reaction. Only choose the foods and nutrients and juices that give your body the essentials to be the best it can be. Remember that everything is energy and every food you consume has either a positive or negative net energy effect.

Health can be effortless, but being sick, miserable, and angry requires an enormous amount of work. When you project good and positive energy out, you will get it back because you'll attract the people who give you good and positive energy back. You'll become a magnet for that positive energy. By the end of the day instead of being exhausted, you'll know the exhilaration of a day well lived and look forward to getting up the next day to continue building your life around this positive interaction with others.

That's a positive way of looking at the day. You surrender the tension and the feeling of guilt about what you didn't accomplish because you're a human being who is in the process of self-discovery. Every day's lesson—positive or negative—is there to teach you something. You learn your lessons one at a time, and by doing so you don't have to repeat that lesson.

Too often a lesson has to be repeated numerous times to be learned —if it ever is learned at all. Think of your situation not as crisis but as a growth process and an opportunity to surrender your old ways. Free yourself to go forward in life and you change the significance of the crisis. You're no longer a victim. You're liberated. A person who doesn't learn the lesson becomes a victim, but the person who does is liberated and ready to experience another step in life.

Clear your mind and bliss will follow. Clear your mind of all preconceived notions. When you clear your mind, the only thing you can have is a blissful state. You can experience it when you're alone with your pet or you're out some place in nature. When you're watching a sunset, a waterfall, or the waves on the ocean, your mind is free of every place except being present in that moment. Keep freeing the mind of old thoughts and ideas that interfere with the bliss. Every time an old thought intrudes, make yourself aware that thought is present and surrender it. We don't need to prove everything in life. We don't have to prove faith, love, and friendship. We feel it. Don't try to prove your value as a human being.

Being a positive, caring, loving, nurturing, compassionate individual is manifesting the highest ideals of life. People will either see that or they won't, and if they don't see it you're around the wrong people. Instead of trying to convince those people of who you are, find other people who will appreciate you. The people who need to make you over in their image are insecure and don't really care about who you truly are. Get rid of those people; you don't need them in your life. When you no longer live your life based upon someone else's preconceived notion of who you are, you free yourself.

It is only after you free yourself that you discover your free will—then Everything Is Possible! Remember that pleasure expands, whereas pain constricts. Look for pleasure in life. Give yourself pleasure in whatever way you want, and don't apologize for it. Discover how much more expansive you are because pleasure resonates all those chakras and all that life energy. Your chi starts to open up and move.

As it moves, other energies will resonate with it, and you'll feel free as your whole body changes. Fear constricts our bodies. Our constriction shows in how we walk and carry ourselves throughout life, the result of our highly conditioned self. Free your mind and pleasure follows. Free your body and pleasure follows. Free your mind, body, and spirit, and bliss follows.

Don't be afraid to start with the raw materials of life. Start with an open mind and open consciousness. Don't be afraid to create something from scratch with your unique identity at the center. When you create anything that's uniquely your own, chances are you'll be happy with it. You'll own it. You may have to do that something many times to get it right, but striving with good intention and right energy and clear vision until you get it right means that each time you make a mistake you will learn from the mistake. The mistake is not something to fear or be angry about, it's merely a learning opportunity! A guidance mechanism to greater clarity. Master the process step by step until one day it becomes easy. It becomes part of you because you own it. It becomes the fabric of your being because you put it together for yourself.

Right now we keep wearing everybody else's hand-me-downs. Whole cultures and nations putting on hand-me-downs as if one size fits all, but it doesn't. We have to make life our own. Instead of being at the forefront of your life, you hide in its shadow. Instead of hiding, honor life by trying to master every single possibility that you can. Think of all the things you could do if you simply allowed yourself the opportunity to believe you could. Richard Bach, author of *Jonathan Livingston Seagull,* said, "Argue for your limitations and sure enough they are yours." A conditioned mind tells you that you can't do something, so that becomes real to you. You can do anything that you want to do. All it takes is first having the courage to visualize it. Once you visualize it you can master it. You can create it. You can do it.

Experiment with your life. As Eleanor Roosevelt said, "Life is a daring adventure or it is nothing." Try things that are totally different. Break the mold that you've been living in and watch how you feel. We live our lives as though we're a butterfly in someone's cupped hands getting brief glances of light and wisps of air. Open those hands and you're free to fly anywhere. Experiment in life and don't restrict yourself by listening to someone else telling you what you can or cannot experiment with. Experiment a little bit every day. Go to different places and talk with different people. Be open to new experiences and break the routine you've gotten yourself into. Break your trance. Shatter your patterns. Deconstruct your habits and construct a new you.

If you don't break the routine, you're not going to do anything new. Reorganize your day so that everything is there for you when you need it. Don't focus on the problems; focus on the solutions. Too many people always focus on why something can't be done. When they tell you that you can't do something, what they're really saying is you can't do something because they wouldn't even attempt to do it. Still other people want you to do things the way they see fit. They act like a savior rescuing you so they can take the credit for whatever you do. The moment you believe you can't do something, you won't. The moment you believe you're limited, you become limited. These are all artificial constructs. They're not real. Like power, they are an illusion. Examine all the ways you've given other people power over your life. Take back that power and start to make your own choices. Don't hesitate or equivocate.

There is never absolute certainty or absolute security—don't wait for it. Uncertainties and fears are never completely assuaged, and you can rarely have absolute confidence you won't make a mistake. If you wait for certainty and security, you'll never do anything in your life. On occasion someone else will falsely give you the confidence and assurance that you're making the right choice, but often you discover it was the wrong choice after all. So remember to listen to your own counsel instead of seeking outside yourself.

Free yourself from all of your limitations and you'll realize how much power you have as an individual. Don't hesitate. Do things without certainty. If something doesn't work out, then you will have learned a lesson and that will make you a stronger and wiser human being. Think of the great musicians, painters, scientists, and athletes who never would have been great at anything if they didn't have the patience to master their craft. Most of us get impatient. Develop patience. Everything done right in life requires patience—a *lot* of patience. Michael Jordan had to miss hundreds of thousands of shots before he mastered the game of basketball. But even as a master he still missed 50 percent of the time. Remember that mistakes lead to mastery.

We're living in a society based upon a great deal of illusion. The idea that living in a bigger house in the suburbs means that you're happier than someone living in a medium house in the suburbs is an illusion. A person living in a penthouse in New York City isn't necessarily any happier, smarter, or more acceptable than anyone else. Getting on the cover of *People* magazine as one of the fifty most beautiful people in America doesn't mean that you're more beautiful than anyone else. That's an illusion. Eating the standard American diet means you're going to be healthy? Wrong. We are inundated with mass media conditionings that are just plain wrong. People have to wake up.

You have to look honestly and objectively at how you have participated in such illusions so you can get to the reality behind them and redirect your life. You need to realize it's time to give up the false beliefs that these illusions perpetuate so you can change. It's now or it's never. And if it's never, then your life will just be more of the same. It's your choice.

So take a look at your life today. Look in the mirror. This is as good as you're ever going to look and feel if you don't do something about it, because nothing gets better on its own. We have to take control of everything in our life and create balance. From balance comes harmony. From harmony comes bliss. When you have harmony, bliss, and balance, you surrender disease, conflict, and anxiety. Don't wait for a crisis to wake up. Pay attention now. What areas of your life are you not honoring? Only you can answer that for yourself, and only you can arrange pieces of your life's puzzle in a way that will bring you joy and enable you to share that joy with others. Remember, DON'T HESITATE—START NOW. Set a new course for your life and realize your destiny will be determined by every choice you make from today forward. Own that power. Honor the life that you deeply desire to live and let no illusion stand in your way.

🌿

CHAPTER SEVENTEEN

What Has Love Got to Do with It?

oday there is an increasingly widespread but unfounded perception that we are merely human beings who have been wrongly conditioned in different aspects of our lives. It is a reductionist belief that finds its roots in early Western psychology and social critical thinking. While past conditioning, beginning from birth and proceeding through the different stages of life, does greatly define our limitations, it is only one component of a larger equation. This chapter offers a new understanding, a new equation for comprehending the various elements that shape the ways we think, feel, and act. An integral constituent in the equation is love. So what does love have to do with whether we spiritually develop and grow or not?

We can begin by exploring our fixed conditional beliefs and values. Is everything that we have been taught by family, teachers, religion, and other institutions correct or not? Many beliefs and values we have learned may be healthy and constructive, while others may be very detrimental and barriers for discovering our authentic self. Even having relatively healthy fixed beliefs does not guarantee they will lead to your living an authentic, healthy life.

Fixed, conditioned beliefs that are passed down through tradition only account for a part of our internal psychological makeup.

My experience with counseling numerous people over the past three decades has convinced me that a significant factor in what determines a person's personal sense of completeness and ability to share intimacy, love, and happiness is related to an understanding of his or her individual life energy. Successful, content people are those who have been able to transition from focusing on the downside of their personality to the upside of their uniqueness that enables them to live authentically. Part of this skill involves being able to disconnect from playing out energies that are in conflict or foreign to our deeper nature.

We realize how crucial understanding our particular life energy is when we see that how our life unfolds is so strongly determined by whether or not we have embraced our proper life energy. There are seven primary life energy types. Individuals who are the natural leaders in a culture can be categorized as Dynamic Aggressives. They perceive themselves as leaders in everything. They are the people who build major multinational corporations and who are sought after for orchestrating successful business ventures. They enable things to happen that few others are capable of. Dynamic Aggressives are reluctant to stand up against other Dynamic Aggressives. They associate and collaborate together; they emulate one another. They construct exclusive communities for themselves and their families.

Next is a group called the Dynamic Assertives. Some examples of this group might include Martin Luther King, Jr., Gandhi, and Ralph Nader. These are individuals who naturally assert the energy and power they possess from a greater perspective of consciousness in order to address the inequalities and imbalances in society. Moreover, they possess a charisma that attracts others. Only the Dynamic Assertive is able to counter the sheer power of a Dynamic Aggressive. The nature of humanity as a whole and the universe itself is not imperfect, but contains a balancing of forces. There is a balance between Dynamic Aggressives and Dynamic Assertives since the latter has the courage to challenge the former.

There are only a small number of Dynamic Assertives in the world. How many Thomas Jeffersons, Nelson Mandelas, Spinozas and Kants, or Dalai Lamas have we had? There have been many people throughout history who have tried to emulate the caliber of these luminaries but it is extremely rare for someone to possess their true spirit unless they are Dynamic Assertives themselves. All the great minds throughout history who have been committed to sacrifice in order to challenge the status quo have been Dynamic Assertives. There have been as many women as men who have had this life energy; for example, Rachel Carson, Barbara Seaman, and Alice Paul were all Dynamic Assertives.

Then there is a group called Dynamic Supportives. These are wonderful, loving individuals who serve as society's coaches. They are easy to be around because you immediately find yourself at ease in their company. You might say they feel like a well-worn shoe. It is their natural inclination to encourage, inspire, and motivate others. They are less critical or judgmental. Among the seven different life energies, the Dynamic Supportives are the ones most likely to encourage you to be the best you can be. They are the ones who will accept you unconditionally—flaws, foibles, and all. While they are not ignorant of other's limitations, they simultaneously see the perfection of your spirit and your life's magnificence and potential. Dynamic Supportives often pursue helping professions such as psychology, teaching, and medicine.

These are the three dynamic energies. I refer to them as dynamic because they are magnificent in the way they project their energy. They will send out a wave of energy to those around them that feels unstoppable.

Next there are three energies that are characterized as adaptive. First are the Adaptive Aggressives. These are society's facilitators and multitaskers. On the positive side, these people can undertake many different projects and assure they will be completed. On the downside, they have the potential to be manipulative and are capable of using others for their own personal advantage. If you have a weakness, an Adaptive Aggressive will zoom in on it immediately and find a way to benefit from it.

The second adaptive energy manifests in the Adaptive Assertives, who have adapted to the status quo. Adaptive Assertives are also the problem-solvers. They are society's engineers and computer geeks. They find their excitement in figuring out solutions others are unable to answer. If you confront a technical difficulty with an appliance or your computer, these are the people who are thrilled to be asked for assistance. Can you imagine a society that did not have Adaptive Assertives to correct all our mistakes and assure us that everything functions properly?

The third adaptive group is probably the largest single life energy, comprising almost 80 percent of the population in the world, and throughout history. These are the Adaptive Supportives, the people who are most comfortable adhering to a single belief. They live almost a monolithic and monotheistic existence. Drew Westen, a professor of political psychology at Emory University, has studied voting habits extensively. His research finds that approximately 80 to 85 percent of the American population votes emotionally on their political party belief system without any critical examination of the candidates' issues and personal characteristics. This large percentage of the population are the Adaptive Supportives. Whether they are Democrat or Republican, they have been so their entire lives and are not likely to alter their belief system.

Frequently when I am providing political and social commentary on my radio program, I make reference to a dynamic that abides throughout the nation that I call "watching Katrina." I use this expression to refer to a particular mentality that clearly sees a crisis looming on the horizon but is unwilling to act accordingly until after the storm strikes. Fundamental change scares these people. What is especially sad is that these are all the hard working, middle-class citizens of every nation who are often forgotten by corporate and political leaders until election time approaches or until they are needed for the benefit of someone else. They become the economic slaves who will adapt to any environment that is presented to them as long as they feel safe and secure.

Adaptive Supportives do not have large circles of friends, but they are extremely loyal to those they do have. They don't like to create waves, and in this respect may seem to appear passive. Television and sports are very important in their lives because they can identify easily with soap operas, Oprah, or allegiance to the hometown sports team. This is their way of experiencing the world without leaving their homes. Dynamic life energies, on the other hand, need to experience the world directly, relying less on the technological medium.

Finally, there is the seventh group called Creative Assertives, who in many ways stand apart from the other life energies. These are society's artists who live in ways contrary to the acceptable norm. Creative Assertives will sacrifice everything for their work and their art. The sensitivities of Creative Assertives are high and so they are compelled to take to the streets to demonstrate for honorable causes, such as to ban pesticides or oppose war. In fact, you will usually see Creative Assertives as the dominant life energy in demonstrations. Emotionally they are very impressionable and sensitive; therefore they need to be approached with great understanding because they are frequently misjudged.

So how do we determine whether we are living the right energy or not? We feel this at the heart level—the feeling that what we do is a true expression of ourself. We will be free from nagging frustrations that there are other desires and ambitions unfilled. I have met people who are Adaptive Supportives but who have attempted to be leaders; however, Adaptive Supportives do not make powerful leaders because their disposition is often a nervous one. They are the group that is most affected with suffering from anxiety disorders because when Adaptive Supportives are placed in a situation that is uncomfortable to them, they will pretend to be fine, which has an unhealthy effect on their bodies and minds.

Conversely, a dynamic person who has been conditioned to be adaptive will experience depression and anxiety as well. For example, dynamic children raised by parents to be adaptive—taught not to stand out from the crowd, to keep their ideas to themselves, avoid risk-taking, not to trust people because the world is dangerous—live in fear of failing and struggle with their heart's desire to do exactly the opposite from their conditioning. By holding back their natural inclination, their energies get blocked, leading to anxiety-related illnesses.

We've been led to believe through our upbringing and culture that our circumstances determine the outcome of our existence. I believe this perception is completely wrong. If you have the best schooling, socially acceptable friendships, have never been abused or denied anything, and have had lots of parental support, it does not guarantee that you will succeed in life. On the other hand, if you grew up in an abusive family and a violent neighborhood with terrible school systems, there are still plenty of opportunities for you to overcome the limitations of your background to fulfill your life's purpose.

When we take the time to focus on what we really want to accomplish in life and on our essential needs, and we learn to surrender what is necessary to achieve our goals, we will manifest our natural life energy. Energy, like intimacy, is not found by seeking it outside of ourselves. We manifest it. Although we have been led to believe that we must hunt for it out in the world, this is erroneous thinking. You cannot simply enroll in a course or retreat, be given a mantra, or sit at the feet of a guru and walk away with intimacy and love. Intimacy, love, and happiness are exclusively the domain of your inner being. It is already there, it has always been, and all we need to do is liberate it. Nevertheless, we must have the courage to surrender our limitations, our false perceptions, and our belief systems in order to complete ourselves.

We can begin by acknowledging that the majority of our feelings and thoughts are conditioned responses. If you wake up in the morning not feeling good about yourself, or you begin your day on a negative note, thinking that nothing positive will happen to you, you need to catch these thoughts and feelings and see them for what they are: nothing but conditioned responses based in the past. By recognizing them as illusions we will expand beyond the boundaries of past circumstances.

Another important element of fulfilling our life's purpose is our ability to harmonize with others. When I can harmonize my energy with someone else, we share a harmonic rhythm together and we can accomplish more than we could by acting alone.

Most of us yearn to be able to find joy in simple things. Have you ever noticed how much effort people have to exert to simply relax? Relaxation is crucial to allowing ourselves to evolve and grow in life. However, if we are constantly frantic, overworked, and neurotic about being responsible for everything and everyone around us, then our true energies cannot vibrate harmoniously. The life force is held in a static mode. Our chakras, our primal energies, become blocked. Taking some time out of our day to reflect upon all the things deserving of our gratitude is essential for letting our life energies to flow freely. I try to show my appreciation for my friends by calling them and expressing my gratitude for them being in my life. Often I will eat in silence, simply feeling appreciative of the food I am eating. These are ways to increase our appreciation.

I expend a lot of energy dealing with many people, so it is necessary for me to be alone to rebalance my energy. Dynamic individuals will appreciate this because dynamics need to occasionally retreat from others. If others do not understand this, they will consider dynamic people as impersonal and aloof. Dynamic personalities also need to realize that they will exhaust themselves if they constantly give while the majority only take. Eventually dynamics can burn themselves out by becoming attached to the energy of those they are trying to help. The art of counseling and aiding others is to act without becoming mentally and emotionally attached to the energies of others.

When I am with sincere friends, we can have fun and be joyful together. There is no need for any of us to prove anything; we accept each other with all of our individual flaws and foibles. On the other hand, when we are with someone who has a constant need to talk and prove something, it is as if that person is not really present with us; they are bringing a draining rather than a sharing energy. Authentic energy is loving, caring, and yet very powerful. It is an energy found in every human being without exception, which you will recognize because it instills a warm vibration throughout your being.

This is the energy we need to be aware of and seek to cultivate. We need to learn to remove whatever it is that impedes us from experiencing this authentic energy.

Most people today focus on trying to be exceptional instead of simply normal. Consider today's athletes—both men and women—who are almost freakishly distorted with excessive muscle mass. We can observe in them an uncontrollable need to compete and win. The image of success chased after today is not the attainment of happiness, love, and caring, but the quest for dominance. This is most evident among financiers who run hedge funds and equity partnerships, among the Wall Street jocks and commodity dealers who manipulate the prices of oil and food. For example, 38 percent of the entire cost of oil is commodity manipulation and yet no politician has tried to present laws to put such manipulation under control.

Being rich today is no longer sufficient. Instead, it is better to be hyper-rich. If everyone is wealthy in your neighborhood, then it is better to stand out and appear even more affluent. If a family down the street has a Lamborghini, then you may believe you should have a Lamborghini and a Maserati. In some individuals, there is an unquenchable thirst to stand out, appear famous, and make others seem insignificant. During the last ten years in the United States we have seen a new class arise: the obsessively rich. So we have individuals who will custom-build giant yachts the size of small ocean liners or purchase Airbus jumbo jets seating several hundred people. But what is the difference if your ship is one hundred feet or five hundred feet in length? The ocean doesn't change, yet the obsessively rich have a need for others to know they possess such monstrosities. Is property really any different if it costs $1 million compared to the home ten miles away valued at $200,000? The answer is "no." It is all a matter of perception.

We are afraid of just being normal because we have transformed normal into something unexciting and unattractive. Yet the most enjoyable people I have in my life are just simple people. They do not confuse the complications of their external life conditions with the simplicity of their eternal bliss. They are easy to listen to because they do not confuse issues. They listen intently to your words and don't misconstrue them. How often have you spoken with a person who takes everything you say out of context and tosses it back at you in a distorted manner? People who live simple, normal lives, on the other hand, avoid such complications.

Normal is in fact the right place to be. When we try to exaggerate our normalcy in order to be accepted, we become caricatures. So many people today are little more than walking social cartoons. We exaggerate because we are afraid of just being normal and living a normal lifestyle.

We should strive to feel compassion for people who have a need to exaggerate because they are the ones most lacking in unconditional love. They do not have such love for themselves so they desperately seek it outside while believing attention is equal to love. However, we only receive love when we let go of our need for attention and open ourselves to our authentic self. Then can we truly connect with another person's energy and find a synergy with that person.

Try to start each day with the thought, *My life is important. If people cannot accept me just for being who I am, that is okay. It is their loss, not mine.* Commit yourself to the decision that you will not exaggerate who you are as a means to run after others. Don't chase after love, because love cannot be forced, demanded, or hunted down. If you think sex can be a tool for securing love, you will fail. So many people believe that sex equals commitment and commitment equals relationship and security. I believe this argument is specious. You will just have a lot of sex without real love. This only leads to frustration and eventually to anger, guilt, and resentment because you have fooled yourself and used others. It would have been easier for you to discover love by opening up to your authentic self.

Remember that all love comes from you. All intimacy originates with you. You can share the love and intimacy you have with another, but do not expect to receive it from someone else if you are lacking yourself. You are not an empty shell waiting for someone to fill you up with love and acceptance, making you suddenly feel alive and complete. A huge subtext in modern American culture, and about women in particular, is that we are nobody until we find fulfillment through somebody who loves us. The idea that a woman is incomplete until she is in the presence of a man is a very sexist and misogynist perception that many of our religious and social institutions continue to perpetuate. The last thing the power structure in our society wants is a world full of freethinking, independent women who would speak out against the conflicts, racism, and male domination that continue in so many sectors of our society. Women with greater influence would offer a balance to the dominant alpha males who still control the territories of property, wealth, and ideas. Women would bring a spiritual balance of energy that we have not seen before. There have been isolated times when expressions of women's freethinking have been tolerated, but only to the degree that they didn't threaten the status quo of the prevailing social paradigm.

The next issue that determines whether or not we are expressing our true life energy concerns our need to create a protective zone. When we limit ourselves to the comfort of a protective zone, we can no longer grow. We can still experience the world but those experiences will not contribute to our necessary transformation and growth. We're trying to protect something. We're not only protecting ourselves by staying comfortable, but we're simultaneously protecting the very institutions that define and support the paradigm which in turn creates the illusion of our comforts. If you are an insider in a group of people who share common views, attitudes, and beliefs you cannot disrupt this comfort zone. If you disrupt it, you will no longer feel comfortable or be welcomed in that group-thought.

There is a woman I have known for about twenty-five years who comes from a community that places great importance upon monetary success. She is forty-five years old, married to a professional man, and has three children. An inordinate amount of her attention is focused on accumulating and prizing possessions. She is a good mother, very caring, and loyal to everyone. In fact, she cares in excess and agonizes over everyone's acceptance of her. Consequently she is chronically busy taking care of other people's needs, but never her own. Her authentic self has dried up, as it were. On many occasions I have encouraged her to be the person she was meant to be rather than to live her life through other people but she is terrified of being judged as anything except "a good girl" who doesn't disappoint others. So her self defined by materialist comfort decides to stay within her circle while her authentic self wants to break through and be creative.

On one occasion she said to me, "I know there is so much more to life and so much more to learn, but I am afraid to explore outside of my community." Therein lies the dilemma, since the risk to fulfill her authentic needs might require her to remove herself from everything she has been conditioned to. Do we have the courage to appreciate our life's passages, have gratitude for where we have arrived, but also to embark on a new journey that may disrupt the world we have been devoted to? Very few people have the courage to make that kind of dramatic transition. We have become a nation of passive spectators unable to break through the illusions that hinder growth. It is impossible to find what we truly need in life by being a spectator in a closed zone with other like-minded people.

So how do we find our own way? We can begin by living with a sense of ease and appreciating every moment we are in. Before acting, we should reflect on the likely outcome: what will happen if I act inappropriately or say the wrong thing? We do not find ease and quietude by reacting to everything and everyone around us. Next, we should not personalize our situations and conflicts with others. Nobody is waking up in the morning for the sole purpose of upsetting you. As long as I stay in the moment I am in, my mind is exactly where I am at that moment. If I am projecting my mind into the future or remembering yesterday, I am no longer present. Instead I have locked myself into an internal conflict, trying to resolve the past, which is a challenging but not impossible task. We can't change the past. But we can change how we feel at this moment. I want to feel good, laugh, feel pleasure, and appreciate the small things in life. I want to manifest the very best I can be. I can only do that if I am at ease and remain in the present moment.

To be a model of health, happiness, and joy, bring yourself to the present moment and ask yourself what your options are now. We all have options, so reflect on the positive outcome you want and act only on that. You can begin by forgiving everything that has prevented you from pursuing your full potential. The power of forgiveness is one of the most powerful spiritual tools and virtues in human nature. Forgiveness should come through love. Think of where the world would be if we could forgive, and start anew from that moment forward.

How often have you held back from being joyful because you were focusing your attention on bills to be paid or agonizing over your many responsibilities? During those moments the mind is wrapped around issues you cannot accomplish. Like a chain reaction, the stress of dwelling on debts and problems multiplies, increasing the responsibilities you feel compelled to control. So only look at what you can accomplish. By keeping your mind positive and reflecting upon what you can do at this moment, you will find greater ease in pursuing a task. This is how you achieve self-mastery.

Whatever we wish to do properly and thoroughly must be done with mastery. Our problems lie in that we have mastered the wrong things. We have mastered anger, reactions, and frustration with excellence. We have mastered the ability to close off our emotions from those we seek real intimacy and love with. And we have mastered guilt and blame. These are our accomplishments. When we dwell on these negatives, we are re-creating them in our minds and they then manifest in our lives.

An excellent, simple daily exercise is to relax and breathe deeply without thinking about anything. Deep inhalation relaxes the entire body. Your pulse rate slows down and your blood pressure decreases. All of your muscles relax and you experience a very relaxed state of mind. In contrast to this state, you can try a small experiment by thinking about something unpleasant, that you will be fired tomorrow or have an accident. Notice that your entire body tenses immediately. At the biochemical level we secrete chemicals that stimulate stress and tension throughout our bodies. We do this all the time whenever our thoughts dwell on one problem after another.

Sometimes it is valuable to be able to share our problems with others. But much better is to first come up with a solution to a problem and then approach a friend or partner and say, "I had this happen to me today and I came up with this solution. What would you have come up with?" In this way, we are inviting another person to participate in a positive outcome. Instead of just sharing frustration and helplessness, you are activating a different part of the brain and energy to explore real solutions to a problem. This is how to be proactive and to grow and mature. Problems and crises then become opportunities for expanding ourselves instead of constraining our energy in a state of fear. When our energy is held in stasis, we end up sublimating: drinking, overeating, gambling, complaining, et cetera. This only makes matters worse because we are building new negatives upon old negatives, and that accumulation magnifies and manifests as emotional disturbances and physical illnesses.

We have been led to believe that we only need to change the circumstances of our lives in order to get rid of our problems. But making changes in the external world, such as moving to a new home or different city, will not change the way we perceive ourselves and others. If a problem resides within you, then you have only moved the problem to a new location. If you have a partner you are not pleased with, and if you are also part of the relationship's conflict, then getting rid of that person and finding another will not remove the problem that has been inside you all along. If you are poor and miserable and then come upon an inheritance or other windfall, you will still be miserable. The only difference will be that you will find other ways to express your misery. The lesson is that circumstances in and of themselves are not the only things that need to fundamentally change. What needs to change is your attitude and your perception about yourself in relation to everything and everybody in your life. Of course there are also circumstances that can be improved. So examining your situation is also important for determining whether you avoid change out of fear or not. Very often changing our circumstances can be a great benefit and lead to new life passages.

We should also cease inflating everything in our lives into greater distractions than they are. How often do we make our relationships or occupations distractions? Make a list of everything in your life that you regard as a hassle and are not pleased about. Whatever comes to mind, write it down and then ask yourself what you can do about each item. Is it possible to transform one negative into a positive? If not, can you remove it from your life? Most people are afraid to unclutter their lives of people, circumstances, and possessions. Yet it is very purifying to reach for our real and authentic self and to remove unwanted baggage from our lives. Take a week or two to think about all the clutter that limits your freedom and independence and how you might remove it. Review every person and possession and evaluate their importance to you. If there is a person who you only argue with and there has never been any resolution in the past, then either find a new way to work things out or cease compromising and disconnect yourself from that person. There are people in my family I do not communicate with because there is no authentic communication between us. There is no benefit to allowing someone in my life who demeans me. There is no point to continue arguing and fighting with people if they won't choose to appreciate you in a loving and kind way. If there is no love in communication, there can be no true communication.

Everyone should be honest about what his or her needs are. If you have needs that do not fit into someone else's expectations, then find friends who can honor your unique needs. I am grateful when people are honest, open, and vulnerable with me. A person is most honest when they are most vulnerable. So often people only tell you what they think should be said in order to be accepted. I do not want people to tell me only what I want to hear. I want people to tell me what they believe and feel. I can agree or disagree, but I will not try to change them. Furthermore, I love to see people empowered. I spend a great deal of time with people who are seeking ways to help and improve themselves. Yes, there are those who will not take advantage of the energy offered, but others do, and I have seen individuals completely transformed.

One way we can help ourselves is to stop looking for the temporary fix to our problems. Instead we should be seeking long-term, sustainable solutions. When people feel our pain and fear, they tend to get uncomfortable and want us to get over it as soon as possible, so they encourage us to make short-term choices. Finding long-term solutions involves committing yourself to looking more deeply and comprehensively at your problems. It means spending quality time alone in silence to clearly see the problems facing you and to find ways to resolve them.

The more imbalanced we are, the greater the pain we experience in remedying our problems. I meet many people who resist going through any transformation process because they sense the pain that awaits them. However, pain does not exist until we create it. The pain we worry about, of surrendering those things we are comfortable with in order to embrace a positive solution, is simply fear. Often people will ask me, "How can I possibly make changes, Gary, if I do not know the outcome of what I will change into?" This is where trust and vulnerability come into play. Both are required to open up and allow your authentic energy to become activated in your life. This energy acts as a radar, scanning everything. You cannot lie to your inherent intuitive and spiritual self. All you can do is learn to be sensitive enough to listen to it because the true self will tell you what is right and wrong for you. It can tell you everything if you are open to it. So don't be fearful of the corrections you must make in your life.

Every April in Central Park I start training people for the New York City Marathon. All kinds of people attend. Some are just out of shape, others are obese. Some have high blood pressure and cardiovascular disease, but they believe they can run the marathon. Every person I've ever trained during the past thirty years who committed to the training protocol finished the marathon. I start them with holding the idea that today does not matter because today's body is the total accumulation of everything from yesterday, and starting now we are now shedding all of the limitations that we have gathered: all of the past inactivity, all the wrong choices are being surrendered. So if you are going to go through any discomfort, do not perceive it as negative. That last final pain of release breaks us free and permits a new person to come forward. It is remarkable to see this happening in people who felt it was impossible. That is what is so exhilarating about committing oneself to confidence and vulnerability instead of to the conditioned self.

More often than not the reason we don't venture too far out of our shells is because we're afraid of losing something. Are we afraid of being replaced? If I am afraid of losing my health, then my energy will be contained in my fear. Rather than becoming healthier, I will be empowering my fears and insecurities. The body responds to your thinking as if it's real. So remember there is only room for the present. When you're conscious and focused in a mindful way on this moment there cannot be any fear. There is no father, mother, priest, rabbi, or anyone else saying you can't or you should do anything. You do not need anyone else telling you what you should feel. There is only you and your free will. Only you can find the key to unlocking the power, passion, and pleasure that opens your self to the world. It is like a door that has been closed and suddenly opens. As it opens, your energy starts to flow into your life.

Whenever you are around a person who has experienced the liberated self, you will notice their presence is very light. On the other hand, when you are in the company of someone absorbed in their repressed, conditioned self, there is a turgid, heavy feeling, as if the person is living in a dank cellar of their existence. We can break from that conditioned state by being quiet, discovering our inner balance, and by saying to ourselves, *At this moment I am the only person in my mind. I will not allow my past to control this moment.* Then you have the capacity to make positive choices. It is that simple and it does not require much time. In a heartbeat you can free yourself. By changing your thoughts you have changed you energy.

Something I truly love about life is that every day is brand new. Every day I have an opportunity to think and feel differently and be inspired by each day's uniqueness. What happened yesterday no longer matters. I am not going to bring yesterday's anger, disappointment, or failing into each new day. Today is unique, a new beginning. It is a day to celebrate and offer thanks for being alive. Every day is an opportunity to appreciate who you are. Appreciation comes from opening yourself and becoming vulnerable. When we are hurt, we have difficulty being vulnerable. The feeling of hurt is rigid, and rigidity blocks the heart energy, preventing us from sharing with others. Vulnerability is the opposite; it is soft and malleable, and allows us to be open and honest with ourselves and others.

When you're honest and open to yourself, internal impediments are removed and everything you wish to feel and share will be effortless. If you ask for something from a vantage point of fear, honesty becomes distorted. Fear generates emotional and mental obstacles that hinder our energy's creativity. The consequence is that we end up making torturous efforts to learn something new but find ourselves unable to surrender the causes of those obstacles in the process. We can seek out all kinds of avenues for renewal and spiritual relief, such as spiritual retreats, meetings with a counselor, reading books like *The Secret,* or watching *Oprah* and *Dr. Phil,* but we still remain unhappy. Yes, some of the information offered by these outlets is good and there are many people making an honest effort to provide us with new insights. The problem is that a new insight cannot be assimilated and induce positive change if it is competing with older negative energy that hasn't been surrendered.

The conditioned self and the authentic self cannot coexist with harmony. The authentic self is easily suppressed. For example, we can talk incessantly about openness and love but we may really be talking about our conditioned need, not authentic love. What we reveal in our lives demonstrates whether or not we truly love. Love doesn't injure anyone. It doesn't manipulate and lie. True love and intimacy means being present for another person who chooses to feel our love.

It matters very little what a teacher—spiritual or otherwise—offers us if we approach those insights and guidance with a closed mind and closed heart. You might believe you comprehend, but unless you actualize those insights in your life the teaching will have little positive impact. The only way you can actualize spiritual insights is by committing yourself to feeling and sharing unconditional love, intimacy, and happiness. This means you must get out of your conditioned comfort zone and surrender your conditioned self and illusory beliefs. All of us are imperfect, so accept your imperfections and those of others. Then vibrate that positive energy so your actions are originating from your completeness instead of from a fragmented, dysfunctional self.

We can identify and examine the areas where we need to grow and evolve in order to become a loving, joyful human being. Each of us holds a vast array of values; some permit us to expand and others constrict our growth. It is important to undergo a survey of all our primary beliefs—relationships, family and children, society and politics, money and possessions, religion, lifestyle choices, values of intimacy, caring and giving, and humanity and the environment. Investigate every belief; make a list of the items that work for you, own them, and then surrender those items that generate conflict and restrict your health and well-being. What you are doing is reprogramming your essential hard drive and removing the programming that keeps you from living authentically.

After we have realigned our belief systems, we should seek out individuals we can be in harmony with. Commit yourself to harmonizing with people at a higher level of your being. If spending quality time with a person is effortless and flows with ease, invite that person into your life. Loving relationships do not require any salesmanship to convince others about your honesty and trustworthiness. Those who have a need to sell us these attributes are in almost all cases those who will act exactly the opposite.

When another person sees you as a model of happiness, joy, and love, and that you are not fearful, you are offering a reminder of what is possible in his or her own life. However, often we may also remind them of their repressed anger; what a person does not like about themselves they will reflect back upon you. If you are a happy, open individual then there will be people who will recoil because they dislike you for manifesting what they have convinced themselves they are unable to be. If you are honest and stand up for truth, you will remind people about why they are dishonest. You are mirroring back to them what they are not. That is why so many people felt enmity toward Martin Luther King and Gandhi. Those who sympathized with these leaders shared in their harmonizing natures.

Everyone has a choice. We can do more of the same and meet with the same outcome repeatedly or we can choose a different way that is new, fresh, and authentic. One of the most frequent activities we habitually engage is endless mind chatter. A busy mind constantly dialoguing with itself changes nothing; only self-actualization initiates change. So we should focus on accomplishing things instead of thinking about things. One self-actualized solution is worth a thousand complaints and legions of mental noise about the problems we are unwilling to surrender.

Appraise all of the circumstances in your life that you can change. Then proactively make an effort to change them for the better. Perhaps you are a sixty-year-old woman who has gone through menopause and has gained weight. Your immune system is stressed and often you experience fatigue. You might have more infections such as colds and flus than before, and have difficulty getting restful sleep at night. Muscle mass is breaking down, skin and hair are thinning, and your libido has diminished. While these are normal symptoms for a postmenopausal woman, it doesn't have to be that way. You can make the determination to change. You can change your diet to start eating healthier foods. You can turn to organic products to lessen exposure to environmental toxins, and drink more glasses of fresh fruit and vegetable juice every day. You can say to yourself, *I will cease eating refined carbohydrates and foods that cause inflammation, such as fried foods and meats. I will remove myself from toxic relationships that increase cortisol levels because of the stress they cause. I will exercise every day. I will start that foreign language I have always wanted to learn or study a musical instrument for the first time. I'm going to use those brain cells I've never used before and look for new, healthy relationships. If the rest of the world believes a sixty-year-old body has to look a certain way, I'm going to prove to them my body can look different. I'm not a lemming that is going to get into line and plunge into the ocean with everyone else.*

This is a way to break through barriers that we have adapted to. But it takes discipline, determination, and balance. Try to make every choice from the highest level of your realization and being. We become wise when we allow our inner being to speak and act on our behalf. We have seen how the conditioned self is more often than not dysfunctional, mean-spirited, and manipulative. There is no need to entertain the conditioned self anymore in our lives. When we surrender it we begin to manifest new energy. Yet as we have seen, it cannot be forced—it requires focus, commitment, and determination to unfold. True growth takes root in us as we surrender everything that holds us in fear and prevents positive change. Finally, be confident and trust in the choices you make. There will arrive a day when you will wake up and feel wonderful about everything around you. Then you will realize that every crisis is a new opportunity for spiritual transformation. Every problem and every challenge is a timeless moment for forgiving yourself and the imperfections of others. Then say to yourself, *I accept the world and other people for what they are. Now I am going to expand. I am going to have a breakthrough and be a more enlightened, happier, and healthier person because I am no longer afraid to live in the moment.*